1982

# Hospice
## A Caring Community

# Hospice

## A Caring Community

**Theodore H. Koff**
*University of Arizona*
*Consultant to Hillhaven Hospice*

*with contributions by*
**Betty Koff**
*Pima Community College*
**Sister Teresa M. McIntier**
*Director of Education, Hospice of the Valley*
**John A. Hackley**
*President, Hillhaven Foundation*
**Robert W. Buckingham**
*University of Arizona*

*Foreword by John A. Hackley*

Winthrop Publishers, Inc.          Cambridge, Massachusetts

**Library of Congress Cataloging in Publication Data**

Koff, Theodore H
  Hospice, a caring community.

  Bibliography: p. 181
  Includes index.
  1.  Terminal care.     2.   Terminal care facilities.
I.   Title.
R726.8.K63              362.1'9              79-27552
ISBN  0-87626-331-7 pbk.
      0-87626-332-5 hc.

*Cover design by David Ford*
*Interior design by Pat Torelli*

© 1980 by Winthrop Publishers, Inc.
  17 Dunster Street, Cambridge, Massachusetts 02138

Printed in the United States of America.

10   9   8   7   6   5   4   3   2   1

# *Contents*

v

# Foreword

The advent of hospice proliferation in the United States epitomizes a dramatic evolution in health care in the history of this nation. However, this unprecedented change transcends the unique hospice concept. It affects every profession and every person contributing to medical and health care. For the first time, successful and effective care is not equated with recovery and cure.

Humanitarians will forever be indebted to the early work of Elisabeth Kübler-Ross. In the preface of her most popularized work *On Death and Dying,* she identifies the purpose of her work as ". . . simply an account of a new and challenging opportunity to refocus on the patient as a human being, to include him in dialogues, to learn from him the strengths and weaknesses of our hospital management of patients." [1] It was surely this *opportunity to refocus on the patient as a human being* that so appealed to the long-felt need of the American people.

With the floodgates thrown open by the first work of Kübler-Ross, there emerged countless other experts through whose thought, work, and writings the needs, rights, and care of dying persons became a prominent concern overtly addressed in all quarters of society. Thus, in one brief decade there has evolved an escalation of acceptance, knowledge, sensitivity, and efforts to increase the scope and quality of resources and care for dying persons as well as the more reasonable acceptance of death as a natural part of the life experience.

Given this burgeoning concern for death and dying among the health and helping professions as well as society at large, it is not surprising that organized attention now is being paid to such related subjects as living wills, human organ bequests, funeral and burial fraud, insurance coverage for catastrophic and terminal illness, multifaceted needs of survivors, and humanization of all care, specifically highlighted in the dramatic appeal of the care of the dying.

1. Elisabeth Kübler-Ross, *On Death and Dying* (New York: Macmillan Co., 1969), preface.

It may be coincidental that during this same most recent ten years there has been critical public and governmental concern about the unrestrained spiraling of medical care cost in the United States. Coincidental or not, this concurrent resistance to the excessive costs of health care led very naturally to an examination of the utilization of medical resources and hospital services in all major categories of cases, including care of the terminally ill. What has long been subjectively known has tended to be consistently substantiated by subsequent study. In the traditional settings in which dying persons in the United States ordinarily receive care during the last phase of illness there is a high incidence of unwarranted excessive use of extreme or heroic means or clinical intervention, inhumane employment of life support systems and undue prolongation of physical life.

The examination of customary traditional care available to dying persons or provided them is undeniably abusive in two critical respects. First, generally available traditional care is often inhumane in that it prolongs suffering, extending physical life with total disregard for the quality of that life. It ignores or transgresses the dignity of the individual, and it inflicts unnecessary isolation of the patient from family, home, and friends at a time when they are most needed. "The dying are now more or less automatically removed from their traditional position at protagonists in a communal drama: the deathbed scene. They are whisked away to the medical fortress where machines instead of human beings will be their companions at the last." [2] Second, generally available traditional care is often clinically unsuccessful in that pain is not continuously controlled, the management of accompanying symptoms is inadequate, and there is not true prolongation of life in all its aspects. Additionally, traditional care can be exorbitantly expensive to the patient, his family, the health care delivery system, and ultimately to society as a whole.

The acceptance by society of death and dying as a natural and healthy concern, the demand by the public for immediate improvement in the humanization of health care, and public and governmental concern for appropriate cost containment in health care delivery have united with the simultaneous expansion of knowledge and skill in the care of terminal illness and dying persons to create a determined impetus to identify, evaluate, and establish effective alternative care modes or options for those who are dying.

In the thoughtful search for alternatives to traditional care, dying persons and their families should look for programs that are highly individualized; that respect the dignity and integrity of the total person; and that incorporate the best specialized clinical care possible into an interdisci-

2. Sandol Stoddard, *The Hospice Movement* (Briarcliff Manor, N.Y.: Stein and Day, 1978), p. 6.

plinary, noninstitutional, continuum of care. Such programs should respond not only to the acknowledged medical and care needs of the patient but also to the patient's and the family's complex of interrelated needs, rights, and desires. Such programs should provide sufficiently diverse levels or types of care within the continuum in a sufficiently flexible manner that the most appropriate type or level of care can be made immediately available whenever a patient's condition changes, whether permanently or temporarily. In the American tradition, institutional care should not be seen as the immediate answer to every problem but, rather, be viewed as an integral part of the continuum as a complementary support to an array of home and ambulatory or out-patient levels of care. In any such search for alternatives, it is inevitable that the relatively long British experience in hospice care will provide valuable examples.

The prototype hospice program model to be described satisfies all of the required characteristics and provisions that society and government seem to be seeking in an alternative care option for dying persons and their families. Already in the United States, and elsewhere in North America, there are virtually hundreds of organized efforts to develop hospice programs that are either based on the more comprehensive British model or are reasonably consistent variations of it, reflecting local preferences, understanding, or existing resources. Although there are as yet a meager few operating services self-identified or accepted as hospice programs, the number is substantial for the infancy of the movement, especially in the absence of even modest reimbursement from the major pace-setting third-party resources.

That the classic hospice program model, as it is generally understood, is adjudged to hold great promise as a desirable and effective additional option that the dying person and his/her family may elect for care is unquestionably attested to by the recent meteoric rise in the number of hospice programs, hospice development efforts, and wide public awareness. In 1979 it was reported that the federal government had identified fifty-nine organizations that consider themselves to be providing at least one service, or level of care, employing the hospice concept and seventy-three other organizations or programs that say they are planning to or are in the process of establishing hospices.[3] However, the National Hospice Organization, although a relatively young organization, enjoys a membership of almost one-hundred incorporated organizations that are either offering a hospice service or are well into the development of a hospice program. The National Hospice Organization also enjoys an individual membership of many hundreds of individuals, among whom it

3. *Report to the Congress of the United States by the Comptroller General, Hospice Care—A Growing Concept in the United States,* HRD–79–50, March 6, 1979, page 11, United States General Accounting Office, 441 G Street, N.W., Washington, D.C., 20548.

is estimated that a majority are personally active in an organized hospice interest group or planning body.

The British hospice experience proves that the British model of hospice care effectively serves the needs of dying persons and their families and is a viable approach to terminal care within the British health-care delivery system. What seems equally certain today is that the American public finds the hospice concept and its underlying philosophy strongly appealing and highly compatible with the recognized needs of dying persons and their families. Unfortunately, what is critically needed and regrettably nonexistent as yet is a sufficiently broad and extensive hospice program experience within the context of this country to fully identify the modifications of the existing British model, if any, that are needed to make it effectively translatable to the health-care delivery system of the United States, retaining the durability and viability of the concept within a substantially different national health care system. This may call for adapting administrative procedures without adversely affecting the integrity of the hospice concept, philosophy, and principles.

The absence of prolonged and validated developmental, organizational, and operational experience of an adequate number of hospice programs within the United States creates the companion deficits of knowledge and know-how to which the hundreds of young hospice planning organizations and groups could otherwise turn for reliable, sound, and helpful guidance in the creation of an effective and enduring hospice program of care within the individual community or region. Dr. Theodore H. Koff has been keenly aware of the dilemma facing the countless hospice interest groups. He recognizes in a most insightful way exactly the kinds of help a well-motivated, committed group or organization needs to develop a hospice program of care that is true to the hospice concept, is philosophically sound, patient-family oriented, and able to endure the vicissitudes of an infant program. *Hospice: A Caring Community* is a major contribution to the hospice movement in the United States and an essential aid to the development of an exemplary hospice program of care.

John A. Hackley
*President, Hillhaven Foundation*

# Preface

This book is written for the student of hospice—whether a classroom student or one working in health care. It is hoped that the ideas presented here may establish or reinforce specific commitment by such students to humane care of dying persons. It is specifically related to persons attempting to learn about hospice care so that their knowledge will help develop or evaluate a hospice program or so they will be able to adapt these ideas to other forms of health care.

Opportunities to establish humane care are not the exclusive responsibility of community planners and builders or care providers. If humane care is to become a reality, it must be a commitment in the hearts of a critical mass of our society who will accept nothing less for all who live.

The builders of a hospice program are all members of a society concerned about the quality of life, and it is hoped that this book will guide them to creative programs.

## A Note of Personal Reflection

To be involved in hospice care requires a special investment of self, a very personal involvement. It is good to begin any hospice effort by reflecting on the meaning hospice has for us. We should seek to understand, and permit to mature, the deep personal concern we have for life.

Having heard about hospice for several years, with interest in its potential for caring, the intensity of my own interest was heightened by two personal experiences with death.

The first encounter was with a colleague who, while dying of cancer, wanted to remain at home with his family. In spite of the physical limitations of a handicapped, but loving and caring wife, he was able to die at home. This was not, however, because of any effort on the part of the physician or of the hospital to which he was referred and its staff. In fact, my friend was admonished by his physician to remain in the hospital in order to receive proper care. A new physician was selected, and a caring community designed a home support program that remained intact until my friend's death. This was my first direct involvement with a hospice-like program.

The other experience was with my mother, who also wanted to remain at home during her dying but, because of intensive pain and in the absence of pain control or hospice program, was forced into institutional care. She was out of personal contact with others long before her death.

These experiences hastened my need to know more about hospice so that I could help in the design of programs to help others die an appropriate death.

I dedicate this book to these two persons: Yetta Koff and David Shirley—and to the users and providers of Hillhaven Hospice who have demonstrated to me the real value and potential of hospice care.

## Acknowledgments

Many people assisted me in the preparation of this manuscript. Each contributed caring concern in his or her own special way. They were supportive, critical, and helpful as they edited, typed, wrote, stimulated, or held my hand. Each knows how important he or she is to me, and I thank each one. Alphabetically, they are Joyce Baum, Robert W. Buckingham, Kristine Bursac, Norman Golden, John A. Hackley, Betty Koff, Dale Lupu, Marian Lupu, Sister Teresa McIntier, Deborah Monahan, Jay Roberts, Barbara Sears, Wanda Ward, and Marsha Weinzapfel.

# 1

---

*Introduction*

---

ONE OF THE QUESTIONS frequently asked of people who work in hospice care is, "Can you tell me everything I need to know to develop a hospice?" The idea has caught on with compassionate individuals and groups throughout this country who are exploring hospice care for their own communities, sometimes for the wrong reasons.

It is often tempting to reply by saying, "Hospice is so new there is little to tell you," or "There are no standards or models; everything is in a flux," or "I've worked so hard to gather my information, why don't you do your own work?" These responses are neither rational nor accurate because:

1. Components of hospice care have a long history in our health care system, although under different labels or identities, and frequently have been part of advanced nursing care practices.
2. Standards and models essential to understanding hospice care exist. While these may be in flux and continuing to mature, we know what ought to be part of hospice care as well as what should not be done.
3. The understanding I have of hospice care has been accumulated from the ideas and labors of many colleagues as well as my own efforts. I would not be in a position to share if others had not shared with me. I share willingly and welcome inquiries, for only through continued exploration of ideas can we reach the goals of providing compassionate care of the dying while caring for them as persons.

Are hospice and the care of the dying identical? No, they are not, but hospice care is both the predecessor and successor to the social events that have influenced our attitudes and approaches toward dying.

Hospice care programs for the dying have been in existence prior to the conceptualization of the English hospice program by Dr. Cicely Saunders. Religious communities, ethnic groups, and extended families have banded together to provide home care of their dying members. For the most part, given the choice, people want to die at home, in the presence of loved ones (Rossman & Kissick, 1962). The severe trauma of pain always has been partially reduced by the closeness of loved ones. A feeling of belonging, the absence of aloneness, and abiding faith in the future are based on the tangible evidences of acceptance and love.

It can be contended that the ideas underlying hospice care are not new, but need to be restated because of the absence of their practice in contemporary health care. To understand how and why hospice has become so significant a force in health care today, it is important to look back at some of the influences that have shaped current practices—directions in health care, concerns about the dying, and the history of hospice care. The selection of background or historical material is of necessity limited because a comprehensive backdrop to hospice would have to delve deeply into health care delivery, economics, social philosophy, theology, and public policy at a minimum. The historical selections cited here are but illustrative highlights of a long history and rich literature.

## Related Issues in Health Care Delivery

While David Mechanic reminds us that health care institutions respond to the same forces in society as other social institutions, hospice has especially responded to these major forces. "Social life generally is becoming more technically complicated, more differentiated, and more bureaucratized. There is a growing sense of loss of community, and social relationships are more segmented and less personalized" (Mechanic, 1972). Health care technology has in many situations replaced the personalized relationship and decreased its capacity to develop mechanisms that support and sustain persons who seek and need help. "Yet the helping institutions themselves are responding to these very same social forces and are increasingly less capable of providing these needed services" (Mechanic, 1972).

Mechanic pleads with us to remember that "we must be constantly aware that the need for medical care and provision of it existed before there was any significant health technology. The forces that brought the sick to the early practitioners and the nonliterate to the shaman still exist as they did in earlier times and the recognition of and response to these forces define the nature of a civilized society."

The same technological advances in modern medicine that have enabled us to live longer and in better health have also not permitted us to die an appropriate death. Medical technology, the high cost of hospital care, medical specialization, and the complicated nature of hospital organizations have created a more technically complicated yet depersonalized nature of health care.

The technical successes of modern medicine flow from a variety of sources, among them the increasing understanding of disease etiology and history as well as biochemical breakthroughs leading to the relatively easy availability of superior tools of chemotherapy. These developments, together with a high rate of technological innovation, are manifested in the proliferation of specialties and subspecialties among physicians and institutions. This has led to one of the characteristics of assembly line production: each practitioner performs limited functions on a segment or part of the patient with a high degree of technical proficiency, but within the current practice pattern, mass production has not led to its usual concomitant: the integration of specialized functions. The vertical integration of separate yet integrally related processes is absent. In its stead we have separation by function, fragmentation by process, segregation by payment. (Berki and Heston, 1972)

The needs of the dying person and his or her family are very personal and care of the dying has to be removed from depersonalized, organizational structure and assembly-line characteristics, returned to the family and home setting, and provided the support of an integrated team of health care professionals in a personalized relationship. These are the essential ingredients of hospice care.

Health care in the seventies has also been influenced by the broader social issues of cost containment, cost effectiveness, and the quality of services. There has been a shift in dominance from the provider of services to the recipient, responding to the vocal representations of consumer groups. The patient is seeking avenues of influence over the organization and functioning of the health care system. Inappropriate uses of technological achievements are being challenged, and providers of health care are required to show the benefits of services and the value of expenditures.

The development of hospice is a response to the issue of appropriateness and questions the validity of requiring that people die in the institutional setting when their preference is for death at home. The dying person needs to retain control over life and hegemony over the health care system to influence it to meet his needs.

Ann Somers (1972), in an examination of health care issues for the future, identified five major themes that to a large extent set the stage for the evolution of hospice in our society:

1. The lifestyle of the consumer and problems of health education. She has special reference to an educated society that can select health care providers, maintain good health, understand the complicating factors contributing to poor health, and manage the environment in its own favor.
2. Availability of twenty-four-hour comprehensive care. To achieve this goal a change of emphasis must overcome the fragmentation of care and stress on acute inpatient care. More care should be rendered outside the hospital in less expensive settings, preferably at home, reducing costs and providing comprehensive care. Such care can be delivered only by teams of health professionals, not by physicians practicing alone.
3. Rationalization of the delivery system. Comprehensive care must

be made available to the entire population at the point of actual delivery, and payment for the services must be assured.

4. Redefinition of professional roles to assure personalized care. The worlds—the world of advanced science and technology, sophisticated management, and specialized personnel, and the world of individual freedom, individual responsibility, respect for privacy, and human dignity. Understanding of the holistic nature of health and disease and appreciation of the need of human beings for other human beings must be widely achieved.

5. Free choice, consumer responsibility, and quality control. People have the right to determine the settings in which they live and die and should not be denied appropriate health care if they choose to die at home. Choice has to be reconciled with quality and quality controls and the patient should know the ramifications of alternate practices. Public and professional organizations and individual practitioners must be held accountable for making this choice possible.

The concept of hospice is, then, a caring system, not cure oriented, with services provided by a comprehensive team of practitioners. Care is offered to patient and family in a choice of environments, but especially in the home.

Hospice is both a response to the existing status of health care as well as a stimulus to assist the health care system to respond to changing societal values of humanism, free choice, and consumerism. Hospice is, therefore, the incentive for change as well as the outgrowth of societal change.

Existing hospice programs have reported on the impact of their programs on the health care system. Hospice units within hospitals have provided evidence that improved patient care results when staff provides personalized care to hospice patients. Some physicians have learned the value of the house calls made in conjunction with the care of hospice patients. Others have learned new skills in pain control and palliative care.

Is there reason to believe that hospice will become obsolete when its special contribution becomes commonplace? This is unlikely to happen for a long time because the same forces creating the need for hospice— high cost of hospital care, mechanization of health care delivery, and increase in medical specialization—will continue to grow. Technological discoveries and successes in the battle against illness and other threats to life will increase, creating greater need for a countervailing force on behalf of humanism, patient comfort, and family integrity.

So hospice will survive for as long as medical care continues to become more efficient, more competent, and more complicated, while necessarily remaining inattentive to the personal needs of the patient.

The deep roots of hospice care in our health-care delivery system stem from a long-standing commitment to quality care and improved health services. They are motivated by our American idealism. In fact, there is very little in the idea of hospice care that is new to our society. Yet we are also motivated by a desire for excellence, and in our search to excel we become specialists in technological advances that seem to reject our commitment to humanism and patient care.

One is made humble in reviewing the importance of our current pronouncements about hospice care when we recall the landmark document of Esther Lucille Brown published in 1961 by the Russell Sage Foundation entitled "Newer Dimensions of Patient Care." In a three-part report of her examination of patient care in hospitals Dr. Brown asserts these important ideas in the provision of health care:

- The present philosophy of the health professions stresses restoration of the patient, physically, mentally, and emotionally.
- Once in a hospital the patient seeks emotional reassurance as well as relief from pain and a physical and social environment that is as little upsetting as possible.
- The patient seeks to adopt the hospital emotionally as a temporary "step-family." When the atmosphere is warm and friendly, he tends to feel secure.
- It becomes the therapeutic task of those persons providing care to attempt to discover each patient's expectations and how they can be handled.
- Patients may have difficulty adjusting to the hospital when they consider themselves unnecessarily robbed of independence and opportunities to make personal decisions.
- Individuals develop affection for and gain satisfaction from a long and varied list of things, whether pet animals, machines, personal possessions, or selected fragments of the landscape.
- Two of the most common signs of family life are children and animals. Around them great affection centers. Unfortunately the support of both children and animals is discouraged in hospitals.
- Eating together around a table is one of the symbols of family life. What is served, and how and where it is served, may be of signal importance to the welfare of sick persons.
- The manner in which a patient is received when entering the hospital may have a profound effect upon his or her perception of being welcome as a human being or only the bearer of a disease to be treated.
- Determining visitation by rules rather than individual concern can be other than therapeutic because visits occur in heavy concentrations, often at times inappropriate for the patient.
- "To deprive patients at a time of great emotional vulnerability of members of their family, of things, foods, and amenities that have

particular meaning for them, of social activities that represent play, sociability, and distraction, is widely assumed, although not yet scientifically validated, to make the healing process longer, harder, or less successful. To place patients in situations where their independence, self-respect, and privacy are needlessly violated is nontherapeutic."

Treatment of the total person is coming to be viewed as essential by members of all the medical and health professions. Such treatment, of necessity, demands a knowledge of the patient's psychological, social, and biological aspects.

Dr. Brown talks about the importance of family ethnicity and culture, of the individual's background and history, to the designing of individualized programs of caring. In making these points, she is the observer of the state of the art as well as the interpreter and advocate for change in responses to the human needs of patient, family, and staff.

The profound similarities between the statements of Dr. Brown and the current principles of hospice reinforce the contention that the roots of hospice are deeply intermixed in our health care system and that hospice has a deep foundation in our own society. These similarities add to our understanding of why the hospice concept has been accepted so easily and spread so rapidly. They also help us understand why hospice will not be a passing phenomenon.

In addition to responding to the growing emphasis on humanistic values in health care delivery, developing hospice programs in this country are attuned to an enlightened approach to discussing death and dying by a host of profound thinkers like Kübler-Ross, Feifel, Kastenbaum, Fulton, Kalish, Weisman, Schneidman, Glaser, Strauss, Garfield, and others.

Each of these persons has contributed to a change in values that is helping to dispel the conspiracy of silence that once accompanied dying in our society and to make it possible for the dying person to find an appropriate place in the health care network. It was important that research be conducted to dispel unspoken myths. It was equally important to develop public forums to heighten individual sensitivities to the problems of dealing with dying and death in our society. The work of these writers should be read and understood by providers of hospice care.

*The Meaning of Death* (1959) and *New Meanings of Death* (1977) by Herman Feifel set a broad philosophical base for studying the issues of death in our society. Feifel says that, "in the last analysis all human behavior of consequence is a response to the problems of death." Feifel sees part of the problem of integrating death into our lives as "an impersonal technology which is steadily increasing fragmentation of the family and dismantling rooted neighborhoods and kinship groups" (1977). At the very least, *New Meanings of Death* should be required reading for hospice explorations.

Glaser and Strauss in their seminal research in care of the dying (1965) look at the social consequences of dying for hospital staff as well as for patients and families. Because most people die in hospitals, these writers are concerned with the interaction between patients and hospital staff and argue for a more rational and compassionate response. They recognize that depriving the hospital staff member of the chance to achieve the primary goal of recovery, and with it the highest nursing reward, results in less involvement and effort in patient care. As an alternative, they point out, the nurse could relinquish the prospect of recovery and redirect efforts to "comfort care" as more appropriate for the dying patient.

The most popular writings promoting an openness to dying are those of Elisabeth Kübler-Ross, who has sensitized large groups of health care providers and consumers to care of the dying and has had great impact on the humanizing of that care.

Her book *On Death and Dying* (1969) was a landmark publication because of its expression of outrage about inappropriate care. From her interviews with dying patients, Kübler-Ross developed a description of a five-stage dying process that includes denial, anger, bargaining, depression, and acceptance. In addition to distinguishing these stages, Kübler-Ross has identified typical interpersonal and organizational problems in care of the dying.

Kübler-Ross's work set the stage for the acceptance of hospice care in this country by identifying unmet needs of dying patients and by providing ways to understand and approach the dying patient. She has also provided the link between established hospice programs in England and those interested in developing hospice programs in this country. The modern hospice concept in this country indeed was made real when concerned persons turned to successful programs developed in England for ideas they could use here to create an improved care program for the dying.

## The Hospice Movement

Dr. Cicely Saunders founded the contemporary hospice movement with the opening of St. Christopher's Hospice in England in the summer of 1967. Every operating hospice program opened since then has taken direction from St. Christopher's. The medical director of Hospice, Inc. in New Haven came from St. Christopher's. The planners and key staff members of Royal Victoria Hospital's Palliative Care Hospital visited St. Christopher's for training (Wilson, Ajemian, and Mount, 1978). The Hillhaven Hospice offers "services modeled as closely as possible after the pioneering St. Christopher's Hospice" (Hackley, 1977).

*History
of
Saunders
experience*

Dr. Saunders traces the beginning of St. Christopher's to her experience with a forty-year-old Polish man from the Warsaw ghetto. They met in 1948 in the general surgical ward of a hospital. He was a patient dying of cancer; she was a social worker. Although he was physically comfortable, he was in emotional and spiritual pain. Dr. Saunders tried to provide emotional comfort, and over the course of many visits their friendship deepened. As they talked, the dream arose in Dr. Saunders of building a home for patients like the Polish man. They began to discuss this dream together, what it would offer, how it could be run. He told her, "I want what is in your mind and what is in your heart." A few days before he died, he told Dr. Saunders he had willed £500 so that he could be "a window in your home." That gift marked the inception of the modern hospice (Stoddard, 1977, p. 73).

Over the next nineteen years the £500 for one window grew to £500,000 for a building and program. First, Cicely Saunders added training as a physician to her social work and nursing background. After studying at the Protestant Hospice of St. Luke's in London, Dr. Saunders went to work at St. Joseph's Hospice. There, during the fifties, she refined techniques for controlling pain associated with terminal diseases (Stoddard, 1978). In 1959 she began to plan for the opening of St. Christopher's, and in 1967 St. Christopher's received its first patients (Saunders, 1977).

Although St. Christopher's first combined all the elements of a modern program, it was not the first institution to specialize in care for the dying person, nor was it the first place to be called a hospice. The roots of the modern hospice stretch back to medieval times to hospices, hospitals, and Hotel-Dieu. These facilities were the ancestors of our modern hotels, hospitals, schools, orphanages, monasteries, nursing homes, and hospices. Sandol Stoddard traces these roots in her book *The Hospice Movement* (1978). Early hospices sprang up along the routes of crusaders, pilgrims, and other medieval travelers. They offered shelter to any traveler, well or sick, and to the hungry, the orphaned, the cold, and the needy, as well as to the dying. They were run by religious orders and were widespread; 750 existed in England and 40 in Paris alone (Stoddard, 1978). However, even these medieval hospices were not the first. There was a hospice in Syria in 475 A.D. (Stoddard, 1978). Fabiola, a disciple of St. Jerome, founded one even earlier in Rome to care for travelers returning from Africa (Stoddard, 1978). Whole religious orders, such as the Knights Hospitalers of the Order of St. John in the 1100s, devoted themselves to the care of the traveler, the weary pilgrim, and the sick (Stoddard, 1978). The Knights Hospitalers offered succor to pilgrims throughout Europe. At the height of their activities, they held land and offered shelter in such places as Cyprus, Italy, Germany, and England.

In the 1800s there was again a surge in the growth of charitable services founded to care for the poor, the sick, the orphaned, and the dying. But now, rather than assisting travelers and children, elders and invalids, the dying and the weary all under one roof, each home began to serve the special needs of just one group. In the late 1800s Sister Mary Aikenhead founded a home in Dublin for the dying (Stoddard, 1978). In 1891 William Hoare of the Merchant Bankers of London appealed through *The Times* for money to establish a home for the mortally ill. This home, called the Hostel of God, is still in operation today. Its management was taken over by the Anglican Sisters of the Society of Saint Margaret in 1896, and they continue to run the sixty-bed hospice independent of National Health Service aid (Anon., 1974).

In 1906 the English Sisters of Charity established St. Joseph's Hospice (Stoddard, 1978), the hospice where Dr. Saunders refined her methods of pain control. In France Madame Garnier organized the Women of Calvary, who founded houses to care for the destitute dying in Paris (1874), St. Etienne (1875), Marseilles (1881), and Roven (1891).

On the other side of the Atlantic the need for care for dying patients was no less pressing. Mrs. Catherine McParlan led a group of Irish Catholic laywomen to establish the House of Calvary in lower Manhattan, New York City. Founded in 1899, it continues today on a new site as Calvary Hospital. Calvary patients have been served by the Dominican Sisters of Blauvelt, the Dominican Sisters of the Sick Poor, and by the Little Company of Mary. Another Dominican order, the Hawthorne Dominicans, founded by Rose Hawthorne Lathrop in 1900, also has a long history of specialized service to dying patients. The order established and still operates seven homes for the terminally ill in Hawthorne, N.Y.; New York City; Philadelphia; Fall River, Mass.; Atlanta; St. Paul; and Cleveland.

Whether called home, hospital, hostel, or hospice, these early institutions were the ancestors of the modern hospice. They nurtured the skills of caring and of hospitality for a group of people practically abandoned by twentieth-century medical developments. They contributed to the modern hospice a loving concern for the special pilgrimage called dying.

But it takes more than the hospitality of the Knights Hospitaler and more than the singular attention to the incurable of the Sisters of the Little Company of Mary to make a complete modern hospice. These older elements *plus* modern pain control, care for the entire family, bereavement counseling, coordinated day and home services, and multidisciplinary teams, must all be brought together—as Dr. Saunders first did at St. Christopher's—to create a modern hospice.

Even before St. Christopher's had opened, Dr. Saunders began to sow the seed of the modern hospice idea and found fertile ground in the United States. Professionals who had individually realized that more could and must be done for dying patients had begun to raise their voices and join together. The Foundation of Thanatology in New York, Ars Moriendi in

Philadelphia, and Equinox in Boston sponsored large conferences on the problems of dying (Foster, Wald, and Wald, 1978). Thus, when Dr. Saunders arrived in New Haven, Connecticut in 1963 to speak to a group of clergy, nurses, doctors, social workers, and students at Yale-New Haven Medical Center, she found a group prepared and eager to learn about a new model and philosophy of care (Foster, Wald, and Wald, 1978).

This talk touched off the planning for a hospice in Connecticut, the hospice that led to the establishment of the idea in the United States. Inspired by Dr. Saunders, a group at Yale determined to bring hospice to their community. Henry Wald surveyed the needs of New Haven and laid out in 1968 the initial plans for a hospice there. Members of the group began to visit St. Christopher's to learn firsthand the principles of hospice care. In 1971 the group incorporated as Hospice, Inc. Several foundations gave grants for community education and development, and in 1973 Dr. Sylvia Lack agreed to come from her post at St. Christopher's to become medical director (Stoddard, 1978). One of her first duties was to seek a demonstration grant from the National Cancer Institute. A three-year grant was eventually received, and Hospice, Inc. began offering home care to patients in March, 1974 (Lack, 1978). A forty-four-bed inpatient facility is scheduled to open in 1980.

Just as Hospice, Inc. was getting off the ground, a conference in Montreal set the stage for the second North American hospice-type program. After participating in a panel discussion on death and dying in February 1973, Dr. Balfour Mount of the Royal Victoria Hospital in Montreal resolved to do more for the dying patients under his care (Wilson, Ajemian, and Mount, 1978). The Ad Hoc Committee on Thanatology was organized at the hospital. Receipt of a $2,000 research grant from McGill University set planning in motion. The committee presented its findings in the fall of 1973 and received a further planning grant of $100,000 from a private donor. Dr. Kübler-Ross came to speak, giving further inspiration to the efforts, and several staff members interned at St. Christopher's. After extensive planning, a twelve-bed unit within the hospital itself was opened in January of 1975 (Wilson, Ajemian, and Mount, 1978).

On the other side of the continent, at almost the same time, the second U.S. hospice group was forming. In 1974 a psychiatrist, a clergyman, and a homemaker met to begin Hospice of Marin, in Marin County, California (Lamers, 1976). Again, planning, research, and community education preceded the opening of the program. In 1975, after unsuccessfully soliciting support from a variety of charitable foundations, the planning group decided to forego an inpatient facility and begin with a home-care program alone. Hospice of Marin received a license as a home health agency and began serving patients in early 1976 (Lamers, 1978).

Hospice, Inc., Royal Victoria Palliative Care Service, and Hospice of Marin all are modeled after the principles of St. Christopher's, but none is yet quite a hospice in the fullest sense. Hospice, Inc. and Hospice of Marin lack inpatient facilities. The Palliative Care Service lacks an autonomous setting and community. The first complete, freestanding hospice in North America had its start in the same manner as the other hospices: the personal experiences of a few community people inspired them to seek better care for their dying neighbors and friends. In Tucson, Arizona, that search again discovered the hospice concept and resulted in the desire to establish a hospice, this one to be known as Hillhaven Hospice. In 1975 several Tucsonans approached Hillhaven Foundation of Tacoma, Washington to discuss the need for a hospice and plans to establish one. The foundation agreed to become a sponsor, and a full-service, thirty-nine-bed hospice opened in April, 1977 (Hackley, 1977).

Up to 1976 hospice was known to only a few in the United States, and programs that did exist were the result of community leaders' having acted upon direly felt needs. In 1976 the movement blossomed. The National Cancer Institute announced its intention to fund three demonstration programs, and The National Hospice Organization formed to facilitate the exchange of information. Conferences were held, and articles began to appear. In 1971 one group in New Haven planned a hospice. By the autumn of 1978, nearly a hundred and fifty groups in the United States had active plans, and thirty hospices had been built in England.

A General Accounting Office (GAO) report prepared at the request of three U.S. senators reviewed and provided information on existing hospice programs in the United States. It reported that fifty-nine organizations considered themselves to be providing at least one service employing the hospice concept; seventy-three others said they were planning or in the process of establishing hospices (GAO, 1979).

The following table shows the number of operating hospices in the United States and their tax status by type of inpatient facility as of September, 1978.

Some hospice programs offer only counseling services to patients in hospitals, at home, in nursing homes, or wherever they may be. Others provide a hospice team in an existing hospital or nursing home. The main thrust at this time is toward home-care programs offering a full range of services, twenty-four-hour-a-day calls, and bereavement services. Few hospices offer a full range of freestanding inpatient care plus home health services.

Since hospice is a comprehensive program of care for those persons with terminal illness for whom active therapeutic treatment is no longer being pursued nor is deemed appropriate, its emphasis is on care rather than cure, and comfort rather than rehabilitation. Hospice care involves the patient and family as the unit of care, with emphasis on control of symptoms under medical direction. The care extends through the bereavement period. Hospice is a concept, not an institution in and of itself.

**Table 1-1** Operating Hospice Programs in the United States

| Type of Facility | For Profit | Nonprofit Corporation | Nonprofit not Incorporated | Total |
|---|---|---|---|---|
| Freestanding | — | 3 [1] | 2 [2] | 5 |
| Hospital | 4 | 19 | 1 | 24 |
| Skilled Nursing Facility | — | 1 | — | 1 |
| Health Maintenance Organization | — | — | 2 | 2 |
| No Inpatient Facility | — | 26 | 1 | 27 |
| TOTAL | 4 | 49 | 6 | 59 |

[1] One of the three freestanding facilities was under construction at the time data was collected.
[2] One of these facilities is a joint venture between two hospitals, and the other is a state demonstration project.

*Source·* U.S. General Accounting Office, *Hospice Care—A Growing Concept* (Washington, D.C.: Government Printing Office, 1979).

Hospice care is defined from the dying person's perspective in terms of individual needs rather than on the system of medical knowledge (Agich, 1978).

Our health care system can be classified as encompassing acute and chronic care. Acute care is characterized by short-stay hospitalization such as that given in response to infectious disease and/or life threatening illness. Chronic care has been identified as long-term care or the care given to mitigate the effects of a chronic illness.

The difference between the acute and the chronic care systems is obviously not related only to the number of days during which care is needed. The real essence of the difference between the systems is related to the expectation a patient using either of them has for the future. Such expectations reflect and are reflected by staff behavior and differing expectations for the patient. A person is admitted to a hospital with expectations regarding the ability of the hospital to rescue life and restore health. These are not the same expectations as those of long-term care, which responds to the needs of the chronically ill who often anticipate neither cure nor total improvement. Obviously there are still different expectations for hospice, where the expectations are for palliative care or symptomatic treatment. Surely these expectations merit partnership with those for acute and chronic care as defining an emerging third level of care.

A GAO 1979 report noted that:

There is no standard definition of what a hospice is or what services an organization must provide to be considered a hospice. However, it is generally agreed that the hospice concept in the United States is a program of care in which an organized interdisciplinary team systematically provides palliative care (medical relief of pain) and supportive services to patients dying from terminal illness. The team also assists the patient's family in making the necessary adjustment to the patient's illlness and death. The program's objective is to make the patient's remaining days as comfortable and meaningful as possible and to help the family cope with the stress.

The National Hospice Organization was incorporated in 1978 to:

Promote the principles of the Hospice concept and the program of care for the terminally ill and their families among the general public and professionals; to act as a clearing house serving the professionals involved in, committed to, and providing services within the principles of the Hospice program of care; to sponsor national symposia, conferences, and workshops throughout the United States to develop and promote ideals of Hospice care; to provide technical assistance to emerging Hospice organizations and Hospices throughout the United States; to provide a mechanism for the monitoring of health programs and legislation relative to the Hospice movement and the needs of the terminally ill and their families. (National Hospice Organization, 1979)

The National Hospice Organization in its document "Hospice Principles and Standards" (Feb. 23, 1979) defines hospice program of care as follows:

Hospice is a coordinated program of palliative and supportive care (physical, psychological, social and spiritual) for dying persons and their families which is provided by an interdisciplinary team of professionals and volunteers under a central administration.
This care is available 24 hours a day, seven days a week. Admission is on the basis of patient and family need. Hospice care continues into bereavement.

In the same document (Hospice Principles and Standards, 1979) the National Hospice Organization states its philosophy of hospice care as follows:

Dying is a normal process whether or not resulting from disease.
Hospice exists neither to hasten nor to postpone death. Rather Hospice exists to affirm "life"—by providing support and care for those

in the last phases of incurable disease so that they can live as fully and comfortably as possible.

Hospice promotes the formation of caring communities that are sensitive to the needs of patients and their families at this time in their lives so that they may be free to obtain that degree of mental and spiritual preparation for death that is satisfactory to them.

## National Hospice Organization

The National Hospice Organization, in its brief history, has both defined the nature of hospice care and contributed to the understanding of the content of hospice programs, their problems and potentials. In this new field of caring, one not yet encumbered by a long history of regulations and tradition, there is the double-edged dilemma of: 1) wanting the time to grow, to experience new ideas, to enable the hospice idea to seek new channels of expression, and 2) concurrently requiring standards and guidelines to assure quality of care and to protect the meaning of hospice care as a unique program of caring for the dying person and family. Obviously hospice cannot both grow unencumbered by constraints and at the same time require the very restrictions it seeks to avoid. Ultimately, the presence of guidelines, state regulations, and professional standards will prevail as in other aspects of health care. Hopefully, this will not curtail creativity and growth, but rather will subject new ideas to the scrutiny of peers, and while slowing down the creative process, will provide greater assurance of the quality of the services. Several states already have passed legislation governing the licensing of hospice programs, but most programs are "licensed as hospitals, home health agencies, skilled nursing facilities and/or psychiatric hospitals" (GAO Report, 1979). Other hospice programs hold no license to provide health care services either because they do not provide services that require license or because the state does not license that level of service.

In the rapid development of hospice care, what should be avoided is the use of the title or concept for purposes other than the provision of hospice care. Regulations and standards will be required to keep the unscrupulous provider of care from using the concept of hospice for anything less than the expected standard.

## Summary

Most hospice programs deal primarily with cancer patients but also include others; some programs deal exclusively with cancer patients. One reason for this is that funding is available for cancer care. Another is that cancer is one of the most prevalent identifiable and fairly predictable illnesses.

Hospice is a revolutionary kind of care that moves the dying back into the home or, when that is not possible, into a homelike setting where patients can surround themselves with their own treasured possessions and friends and family. Hospices are gaining favor in the United States partly because they are an alternative to the isolation of dying persons as well as to the "cure at any cost" syndrome, both frequently the only options offered in acute care hospitals. Hospice also responds to resistance to hospital regulations that often keep families, children, and pets away from patients in time of crisis. But even if hospitals were to relax their regulations regarding visiting and pets, they would not necessarily provide hospice care. Hospice offers a care option that recognizes the slowly emerging wish for death with dignity and the search for alternatives to inappropriate institutionalization.

Students of the dying process have long emphasized the loneliness of the dying person. Not only is he destined to go where no one wants to follow, but the people around him frequently pretend that the journey will not take place. Recent advances in innovative technology are altering the character of dying and compelling us to look more resolutely at death. The impact of an impersonal technology tends to alienate us from traditional moorings and weakens institutional and community supports. It is a historic phenomenon that consciousness of death becomes more acute during periods of social disorganization, as in our present time when individual choice tends to replace automatic conformity to consensual social values. This same death consciousness took place in the early Renaissance, after the breakdown of feudalism. Further undercutting our capacity to integrate personal death is a social system that steadily increases the fragmentation of the family, dismantling rooted neighborhoods and kinship groups. Today the family is essentially nuclear; no longer do we live in a community with uncles and aunts, siblings and cousins, possessing homogeneous values. "Consequently, when death intrudes into our lives, the previously existing institutional and emotional supports to cushion the impact are absent." (Feifel, 1977).

Another circumstance that has made death more difficult to confront is its gradual expulsion from common experience. While direct exposure of children and young adults to death or dying is decreasing because of medical advances, death and dying are given considerable but unrealistic attention in horror films. Death becomes a violent experience when viewed on television or in films. (Feifel, 1977).

In a society that emphasizes the future, to contemplate dying is to state nonverbally that no future exists. "Death is seen as the destroyer of the American dream—the right to life, liberty, and the pursuit of happiness." (Feifel, 1977). All of this points to hostility toward death and a tendency to repudiate it. This outlook may in part explain the generally negative attitude many have toward old age, which frequently precedes death.

## Guidelines in Development of Hospice Programs

Those readers who are developing a hospice program will find in the following pages a statement of hospice principles. These can be used as a road map to keep the effort on the right track as well as a sounding board to determine if all relative issues have been considered.

A principle is a statement of a relationship between two or more concepts or a generalization made from observable events and can be used for determining future action. Concepts are abstractions generated from observable events, a shorthand representation of a variety of facts, or a summarization of a variety of related events.

Principles, as used here, represent the intent to bring together, in a coordinated manner, the observations, experiences, and personal reflections regarding what hospice is and should be in our society.

Without principles, the goals of a hospice program are vague, and the ability to offer hospice care remains elusive. All programs need not be alike nor emulate an existing model. Yet all programs should demonstrate an allegiance to a basic hospice philosophy communicated in this set of principles.

But while principles are necessary and can serve as critical guideposts on the pathway of moral decision making, it may be dangerous to employ them as the only guidepost (Brady, 1978). We should add to the guidepost an ethical signpost that asks us to question how the death experience occurring with the care and support of hospice can become a fully human experience, responding to the human values of each hospice patient.

For purposes of this book, principles of hospice care have been organized as they relate to:

1. *The Person* in need of or utilizing hospice care and those family members and friends who are significant to the individual requiring services.
2. *Control of Symptoms* or guides for assessment and control of symptoms.
3. *The Program and Services* that should be included in hospice.
4. *The Staff* responsible for transmitting the goals and services of hospice to the person and family.
5. *The Hospice Environment* in which inpatient services are provided.
6. *Administration* of the hospice program.

Each of these is presented as a chapter with the full realization that the divisions by chapters, principles, or discussion is often artificial. It is always the ethical signpost of concern for the total human experience that is needed to integrate the disparate parts into a whole.

But before proceeding with the principles of hospice care, it seems appropriate to challenge the reader planning to develop a hospice program to defend his interest in a hospice program and his expectations for it by answering the following questions:

What is your interest in hospice?
Why do you want to develop a hospice program?
Whom have you planned with in the community?
Whom do you represent?
Where will you get your funding?
Is the program getting started because . . .
   . . . of the interest of some individual?
   . . . your community doesn't have a hospice?
   . . . you need a rallying point around which a community can be organized?
   . . . your hospitals have vacant beds with entire wings unused?
   . . . hospice sounds like the solution to poor nursing home care?

All of the reasons cited, and probably many others, have been offered as providing an incentive to initiate a hospice program. All appear to be inappropriate, and the many hospice programs that are moving for the wrong reasons should be realigned, or they are probably destined to fail. Additionally, inadequate programs called hospices present a threat to genuine hospice efforts because communities have not yet developed the sophistication to look beyond the label and appraise the intent and quality of the care.

The basic tenets of hospice care are indeed simple to cite and repeat because of their foundation in the common code of humanism, concern for the quality of life, and reverence for life. This simplicity tends to be deceptive and thereby entraps people into a false assumption that it is easy to develop a hospice program.

We therefore offer this *caveat,* that hospice care is difficult, that it requires substantial commitment from major groups in the community, and that many long, hard, hours of work will be required before a hospice program is realized.

Hospice has become important because there is an absence of the humane hospice values in the current practice of health care and because the growth of humane values in our society at large has set the stage for these expectations.

Hospice cannot overcome pervasive limitations in the delivery of health care, but it has established a new morality in expectations. If hospice can do it, why can't the same quality of services be provided in other levels of care? Hospice has in fact become the teacher of these values:

· The basic regard for the recipient of care.
· Acceptance of death as a natural part of living.

- Consideration of the entire family unit as the patient.
- Sustaining the patient at home for as long as possible.
- Helping the patient assume control over his own life.
- Teaching the patient self-care.
- Reduction or removal of pain and other distressing symptoms.
- Total, not fragmented, care.
- Comprehensive provision of services by an interdisciplinary team.
- Continuity of services after death.

Hospice should only be developed if there is a conviction that hospice care will improve the quality of living for the person who is dying, that the ideals of hospice are in consonance with the values of the sponsoring group, and that there are sufficient persons prepared to assure that the idealism will become part of the functional program.

# 2

---

## *The Person*

---

*Within every person is a distinct and unique being that is unlike any life that has existed or will ever exist again.*

Clark E. Moustakos, 1977

*We have the endless fascination of watching each individual come to terms with his illness in his own way and come along his own path to life's ending. Almost inevitably it is a quiet ending that leaves behind a sense of real fulfillment.*

Cicely Saunders, 1965

THOMAS LEICHT (1978) SAYS that physicians in the past have been taught to investigate illness, to diagnose illness, to cure people of their illness, and to extend life. He advocates the addition of a fifth, most important skill, which is to improve the quality of life of patients. This can be done by redirecting the emphasis of treatment from the disease process to the symptoms that the disease causes in the person. The emphasis needs to be on the person, the quality of the person's life, and maximum fulfillment every day so that the person can enjoy life to its fullest.

By carefully listening to the fears expressed by his patients, Leicht developed an appreciation for hospice care. He organized the many fears expressed to him into the following group he calls "The Seven Fears of Dying."

## The Seven Fears of Dying

The first fear is the fear of the process of dying. Patients are concerned as to whether death will be painful and whether they will be anxious and frightened. They are concerned about their body image. This is especially true of the cancer patient who has lost weight and who when he looks in the mirror and sees his changing image and wonders what is going to happen to his body as death approaches.

Secondly, there is the fear of loss of control. Life-threatening illnesses gradually make patients more dependent. The father can no longer provide for his family, the mother can no longer care for her home and the child can no longer play with his peers. As the disease progresses, we thrust the patient into a health care system which makes the patient and family more dependent. This is especially true in the hospital where we frequently make patients wait in admitting departments and then when they get to the floor, we take their clothes and medications away. We tell them who can visit and when they can be visited. They are told when meals will be served and when they will receive personal care. Patients and families must be allowed to be active participants in the treatment program.

Thirdly, patients fear loss of one's loved ones. They are concerned about what is going to happen to them. Will there be sufficient money to put the children through school? Will my wife have to return to work? How will my family get along in my absence?

*Editor's note:* Readers familiar with the standards of care developed by a task force of the International Work Group on Death, Dying and Bereavement held in January 1978 at Columbia, Maryland, may notice similarities between those standards and the principles described in this volume. The kinship is a natural one, since a number of participants in the task force chaired by Florence S. Wald also made direct and indirect contributions to this book.

The fourth fear comes from a statement by Ted Rosenthal who said, "I never knew what fear was until I saw it in the eyes of the people taking care of me." I cannot over-emphasize the importance of non-verbal communication. Patients read how we are reacting to their illness more clearly than we can imagine.

Fear of isolation is the fifth fear. Patients are fearful of the aloneness of dying. They sense isolation by the frequency of our visits, by the length of our visits, and by our body language. Physicians often have less meaningful things to say as disease progresses and studies have shown that frequently it takes longer for the nurse to answer the bell of a dying patient than the bell of the patient in the next bed who is going to get better.

The sixth fear is that of the unknown. They wonder what can they expect in the way of physical suffering? It is here that one begins to question his faith system and he wonders if there is life after death and if there is, what is it like?

The final fear is that life will have been meaningless. Ted Rosenthal said death is "the time when mind's own camera is forever turned on self." It is the time we look back at our life to see what meaning it has had. Has the world been better because we were part of it? For the person who feels this life has been meaningless, it is important that we help him to identify those positive aspects of his life. If a person feels his life has been meaningless, he then must ask the question why was I created in the first place? This thought can be devastating.*

Hospice, the program of caring, can best be understood by examining some of the critical ideas that deal specifically with the patient. These include:

- Death with dignity.
- Palliative rather than curative care.
- Individuals' control over life.
- The significance of time.
- Elimination of isolation in dying.
- The importance of family.
- Caring for children.

## Death with Dignity

Dignity can be defined as the quality or state of being worthy or esteemed.

The essence of hospice care is in providing the opportunity for the

* Reprinted by permission from *Faith at Work* magazine, April 1979.

dying person to have a sense of worthiness while dying. Although the body is traumatized and shattered by cancer or other diseases, the person must remain intact, be enabled to live throughout the dying process, and maintain a sense of control over his life. Dignity is as much a self-perceived phenomenon as it is a reflected interpretation of the responses of others. Hospice can communicate a sense of the importance and value of the person in spite of ill health. Hospice can also communicate to the person who is not expected to live that defiance of death is neither admirable nor desirable.

**Principle:**    *Enabling a person to die with dignity includes taking whatever measures reduce or eliminate pain and discomfort and always treating the total person, not merely his symptoms. These practices provide security and build trust by focusing on the patient's needs and treating each person as a special and unique being. The dying person is encouraged to express any emotion, without fear of what another may think, and he is helped to die in a way that is appropriate for him, rather than in a way prescribed by others. Permitting death with dignity also means enabling the person and those important to him to practice rituals or to behave in ways in keeping with their culture and/or lifestyle.*

**Discussion:**    It is important that hospice continue both to reinforce the sense of worthiness of the dying person and to avoid communicating disappointment at the person's death. This is not to suggest the absence of regret that the person is dying, and dying of cancer, but since these events are inevitable, all energies should be directed to supporting the individual to an appropriate death.

Cicely Saunders of St. Christopher's Hospice makes the distinction between *care of the dying* and care of the *dying person* because it is the person who is or should be at the center of concern.

Foremost in the concern for dignity should be the ability to control the pain which may be involved, the related discomfort of dying, and the concomitant physical and emotional symptoms of the dying person. A feeling of meaninglessness can be the hardest pain of all for a dying person to bear. Sometimes it is difficult for staff to deal with this. The dying person may find support in different ways. For some, it may be by sensing continued interest in them as people. For others, it may be by spiritual support or by having someone listen and understand.

The dying person deserves the best physical and emotional care. There is no dignity in pain, in incontinence, in nausea, or in the presence of any other manageable symptoms. All of these symptoms rob one of the ability to focus on living.

Each individual is unique, no one person is precisely like another. Because he is not a body part but a whole, total, human being, care should be directed toward the whole person, not the special organ that is receiving the attention. Total care supports the dignity of the dying person as it clearly communicates an appreciation for the person, not the illness, diagnosis, or aberrant behavior or social value of the illness. Total care looks past the diagnosis and facade of illness and attempts to support the person. It also gives the person a vital message—"*You* have value, you are important and worthwhile."

Dignity also means a sense of security in the hospice treatment, a reinforcement of trust demonstrated in the behavior of hospice staff. Staff members must communicate a sense of trust, honesty in their promises, skill in giving care, and involvement and concern with the person receiving care. The casual "I'll be back in a moment," frequently associated with health care providers, must be timed and measured not to exceed the conventional wisdom of "the moment." Staff must be available to respond to the schedule of the hospice patient rather than to organizational schedules.

In a sense, then, hospice staff must defy the organizational imperative that rules are made for staff convenience, not the patient's comfort. Dignity is related to focusing on the needs of the patient and the ability of the patient to demonstrate control over his environment and his dying.

Dignity of the dying person requires a discussion of the meaning of "patient." The word is generally used to identify someone who receives treatment, implying a cure or reduction of the severity of illness. Because this is not an appropriate expectation for the recipient of hospice care, every effort must be made to identify the recipient in a caring, interpersonal role different from that of a patient. Intellectually and emotionally, the role must be made one that emphasizes that the individual, although dependent and weak, is in control and requires, even demands, dignity in life and death.

Respect for dignity also implies permitting, and even enabling, the dying person to feel and experience whatever emotions are appropriate for him, according to his own timetable or schedule. Davidson (1978) supports the premise that denial is an appropriate and inherent part of dignity for some dying persons. Insistence that an individual should "accept his or her fate" is a parochial viewpoint that imposes the helping professional's values on the individual. The ability to deny the stark realities, in spite of the expectations of the caregivers, may be evidence of the strength of the person and his capacity to retain dignity.

People die in the same way that they have lived. An authentic death or an appropriate death is dying in accordance with one's own desires and is congruent with one's life, including cultural practices that may seem strange to those from other backgrounds. It is imperative that hospice staff members support congruity for each individual dying person and his family. In "The Dying Patient's Bill of Rights," there is a statement that sums up the expectations from caretakers of behavior that protects individual dignity: "I have the right to express my feelings and emotions about my approaching death *in my own way*" (AJN, 1975).

## The Dying Patient's Bill of Rights

I have the right to be treated as a living human being until I die.

I have the right to maintain a sense of hopefulness however changing its focus may be.

I have the right to be cared for by those who can maintain a sense of hopefulness, however changing this might be.

I have the right to express my feelings and emotions about my approaching death in my own way.

I have the right to participate in decisions concerning my care.

I have the right to expect continuing medical and nursing attention even though "cure" goals must be changed to "comfort" goals.

I have the right not to die alone.

I have the right to be free from pain.

I have the right to have my questions answered honestly.

I have the right not to be deceived.

I have the right to have help from and for my family in accepting my death.

I have the right to die in peace and dignity.

I have the right to retain my individuality and not be judged for my decisions which may be contrary to beliefs of others.

I have the right to discuss and enlarge my religious and/or spiritual experiences, whatever these may mean to others.

I have the right to expect that the sanctity of the human body will be respected after death.

I have the right to be cared for by caring, sensitive, knowledgeable people who will attempt to understand my needs and will be able to gain some satisfaction in helping me face my death.*

## Palliative versus Curative Care

Curative means that which will restore health; palliative can be defined as mitigating or alleviating symptoms.

In the framework of a cure orientation, the disease is treated. There comes a time, however, when the conclusion must be reached that all efforts to effect the cure of certain persons have been exhausted and nothing else curative can be done. Failure to find a medical cure does not mean, however, that the individual no longer needs care. And caring for another person in the most significant sense is to help him grow and

---

* This Bill of Rights was created at a workshop on "The Terminally Ill Patient and the Helping Person," in Lansing, Michigan, sponsored by the Southwestern Michigan Inservice Education Council and conducted by Amelia J. Barbus, Associate Professor of Nursing, Wayne State University, Detroit. From *American Journal of Nursing* 75 (January 1975): 99. Reprinted with permission.

achieve a sense of fulfillment. Care in the context used here refers to unifying and integrating the dimensions of living and includes those skills that assist the person to become whole (Davidson, 1978).

**Principle:** *Hospice care emphasizes relief of symptoms. When health restoration is no longer possible, care, not cure, is the focus.*

**Discussion:** Care allows a wider scope of action than cure in that it includes ideals and goals in addition to seeking so-called "normal" physiological and psychological function. Among such goals are comfort and ease. Palliation can also be viewed as a hopeful, realistic goal, demonstrating that more can be done to comfort the individual.

The significance of the distinction between palliation and cure is challenged when a palliative care program is introduced into a curative care environment, i.e., hospice care introduced into an acute care (hospital) or long-term care (nursing home) environment. In the curative milieu there are dual goals: curing and caring. These goals are internalized into the structure of the organization, its medical care, its total services and, therefore, the expectations of its clientele. Whatever inconveniences exist—diagnostic testing, a regimented lifestyle, the pain and nuisance of treatment modalities, etc.—are tolerated because they are seen as contributing to generally accepted ends of cure.

In contrast to acute care, the hospice offers care and provision of a sense of well-being. The hospice concept is not a technical skill, procedure, or drug intended to eradicate a specifically diagnosed abnormality. In hospice, care is directed toward an individual and becomes a quality of ministering to that individual, who happens to be sick. While hope must never be withdrawn from any dying person, the care provider should clearly represent a caring environment without representing false or inappropriate expectations.

If there is a unique qualitative difference between cure and care, it would be most genuinely represented by the efforts of the program staff. A palliative care program should minimize the conflict between the concepts of cure and care that torments staff members at other kinds of institutions and permit hospice staff to be completely committed to caring. Achieving this is made more difficult by the frequent pressure imposed by funding sources to demonstrate rehabilitation potential and plans for discharge from the health care environment. Care providers are socialized to view patients in terms of potential for improvement in their health status; written records are expected to reflect this potential as justification for committed supportive payment as well as for subsequent care.

The organizational structure of a hospital or nursing home—its staff and reward systems—prides itself on cure and rescue from near death. Staff in hospice must be focused on caring and must feel none of the pressures for cure. Caring for people near death and assisting people to die appropriately must be sufficient reason for their dedicated effort. There can be no compromise.


## Control

In hospice care, the dying person and his family are encouraged to maintain or regain control over their lives and to use the health care system with few compromises of their own authority.

When individuals are in pain, they lose control over other aspects of their lives in the all-consuming experience of pain. Other symptoms also promote loss of ability to focus and, while not so all-consuming, cause a diminution of independence and reduce options and choices. By treating the disquieting and discomforting symptoms, hospice staff members permit each person to deal with his own dying, family, and life. There is dignity when an individual makes decisions affecting his life. In essence, he, not others, is in the "driver's seat" in making choices affecting his own life.

**Principle:**    *In hospice care, the locus of control must be redirected to the dying patient. When the goals are cure of some diagnosable disease, the patient accepts some limits on his ability to control his life—usually for a limited period of time. There should be few limits placed on the terminally ill patient in controlling aspects of his life.*

**Discussion:**    Control over choices and situations varies with the age of the person, the severity of illness, and the level of the patient's dependency. Very young children, like the old and the very sick, have little control. Generally, there is little reverence shown toward the aged person in our society, and there is less reverence shown to the dying older individual. There is dignity in being revered if it means your wishes and concerns are solicited and respected. Hospice care providers must support those strengths in care for recipients that enable the recipients to assume control over themselves, the environment, and the situation. When organizational rules and policies are made, they must reflect the fact that the policy is for the patient's benefit. Questions that should be asked when any policy is written are: "Who will it benefit?" "Who will it hurt?" and "Who will it affect?"

Hospice care should stress the importance of life control for its patients and be prepared to support individual lifestyles with policies that are flexibly responsive to the needs of the patient and his family. Helping the patient to die at home, rather than in an institutional setting, when that is the patient's choice, is one way of enabling the individual to retain control. Because support of self-determination is an important hospice principle, evidence of its intent must be made clear to the patient and his family. During early interviews and subsequent meetings, hospice staff members should try to learn of each patient's interests, values, and life-style. The questions, "How can hospice help you and your family?" as well as "What special requests do you have that would please you?" should be frequently asked. Subsequently, it is incumbent upon staff to assure that responses are faithful to requests and are, whenever possible, made promptly. There will be requests that cannot be honored; in such situations, a clear explanation of the reason for not honoring the request should be offered.

Requests for special foods, for visitors, for privacy or company can be handled easily, but what about the request for the companionship of a special pet? It is the request for something so outlandish as to be immediately perceived as impossible that really taxes the hospice staff member. When that staff person finds himself or his program saying no instead of yes, it is time to explore what can be done to reverse this.

The ability to invite requests and then to respond affirmatively to them is evidence of regard for the person receiving care and respect for that person's control over his life.

Capacity to exercise control over one's life is obviously an individual variable and must be seen as continuing from earlier life experiences. The dependent person may not seek independence at his death. Independence may be too threatening and create anxiety and pain. Dignity and self-control as a goal for hospice care require that a careful assessment be made of the individual's life situation, including cultural values, with the care provider supporting the person's lifestyle.

## Significance of Time

Each of us who lives will someday die. The hospice patient lives with greater certainty that his end of life is near.

An important principle in hospice care is the appreciation of the significance of time, both for the dying person and the care provider. The patient may be in a race with time—to resolve all the unfinished business of life or to nurture all that life can offer in his remaining time. While the life span of all human beings is limited, the dying person is aware of the close proximity of death. He is realistically aware that each day and every event and experience may be the last. The hospice client should not have to insist upon the urgency of each request nor have to seek special treatment to have the request granted.

**Principle:** *Caregivers must function to perform tasks and give care to fulfill needs "now," avoiding postponement. Hospice care should always* *keep in perspective that any request may offer a last opportunity to care for the person, that any request may be a last request, and that any postponed or unfulfilled request may never be honored.*

**Discussion:**    Work tasks have to be reordered to give priority to the patient. The "I'll do it for you in a minute" syndrome so frequently overheard in health care environments realistically refers to a postponement that is usually much longer than a minute. The hospice environment has to be permeated with a "do it now" response reaction that argues for the earliest response humanly possible. For example:

| Patient | Inappropriate Care Provider's Response | Required Response |
|---|---|---|
| I'd like to talk to my son. | It's late, we can call tomorrow. | Do it now! |
| I'd like to see the chaplain. | He's off today, I'll tell him tomorrow you were asking for him. | Do it now! |
| I haven't had a pizza in years. I'd love one now. | You just finished dinner. I'll ask the chef to get you one tomorrow. | Do it now! |
| I'd like to smell some fresh flowers. | The next time your daughter comes, I'll ask her to bring some. | Do it now! |

In order to achieve the "do it now" response, staff must be oriented to the importance of time and the timely response to the dying person. Beyond that, it is essential that there be sufficient staff available to accommodate the urgency of needs and to have the ability to respond within the expected time frame. Staff members need not feel that they are the only ones capable of responding to requests; they should be ready to use the resources of family and volunteers to enable them to bring the response as quickly as possible. Hospice care should provide a team made up of family members, practitioners in various disciplines, and volunteers who regularly respond to personal needs. In this way, the dying person can choose who will be asked to respond to his different needs. This permits a high degree of freedom and, thereby, ability to exercise control over the environment.

Goals for patient care must be short-range, have great flexibility, and be reviewed frequently. The time frame may be in terms of hours rather than days or weeks, requiring more intimate involvement and more careful observation of the patient and his family.

The urgency of giving a rapid response to the patient's needs can be compared with the timing of the expected response in a hospital emergency situation. In the emergency situation, time is important because of life-threatening events. In hospice care, time is important because of life-nurturing events. Hospice needs quickly to learn as much as possible so that it can offer as much as possible within the time remaining for the patient.

Staff team meetings held on a weekly basis will not be sufficiently responsive in hospice care. Team size must be kept small and membership flexible so that the team can be quickly convened to plan for care. The arrival of a new person in hospice care should signal the immediate assumption of a new planning cycle, rather than waiting to fit that person's needs into an existing schedule.

## Eliminate Isolation in Dying

The fear most frequently expressed by dying persons is that of being deserted. Many cultures prescribe behavior that emphasizes the need for family and/or others to stay with a dying person. Other cultures encourage or insist on the ailing person's withdrawal to die in isolation.

The fear of isolation in dying persons in our society is most critical for the person, socialized to the idea that the "right" death occurs only in the presence of loved ones, who finds himself alone when he senses death is near. However, the assumption should not be made that all persons fear isolation in dying. The desire for steady companionship should be explored with each person.

**Principle:** *The dying person must be assured that he will not be alone, that someone will be with him should that be his desire, and that he will not be forgotten or deserted at death.*

**Discussion:** In spite of recognizing mortality, many individuals go through elaborate rituals to provide continuity to their memory and in that way, to their being. Cemetery headstones, mausoleums, memorials, named buildings, bridges, programs, etc. all provide continuity. The dying person, especially one without close social contacts, fears isolation at death, with no one near to soothe the pain, respond to the crises, or just observe and respect the event.

Somehow, the unobserved death is made less significant because the moment is not shared with loved ones, or those who care. The devaluation of the aged, sick, and dying in our society is manifested in a reduction of meaningful social contacts for the dying person. Friends drop away; the trauma of observing physical deterioration prior to death repels some. The dying person is a symbol of our own mortality, which some of us can accept and some cannot.

The frailty, disability, and severe weakness accompanying the dying process, especially in cancer-caused deaths, results in an inability to control the environment. This can be accompanied by the fear of helplessness, anxiety about choking, incontinence, or the ability to protect oneself in crisis situations such as fire.

In hospice care, the assurance should be given to each person that he will not die in isolation either at home or in the institutional environment.

The resident who for very private and personal reasons wishes to die alone or with only a staff member must be respected. Several anecdotes may help illustrate this point.

An alert and delightfully gregarious seventy-year-old resident made the decision to experience dying alone and independently. During her stay at hospice she often regaled the staff about her exploits.

One night when the nurse was making rounds, she found the woman awake and offered to sit with her. The woman expressed appreciation for the offer but gently asked the nurse to return in a couple of hours. An hour later, however, the nurse again looked in and found the woman had died in the interim. Her facial expression gave evidence of a peaceful death, as there was just a suggestion of a smile on her lips.

Another resident of hospice, a frail but very independent woman, had done all she could for her family. She had come to accept the reality of her approaching death, but her husband was unable to. Frequently he pleaded with her to live and on occasions would cry out in anger, accusing her of not wanting to live. But the woman had set her trajectory, and on the day of her death she told her husband to take a little break and relax in the day room. He was away from her a short time when she quietly and peacefully died.

Hospice care requires that there be a twenty-four-hour-a-day availability of support persons to comfort dying persons and be there when needed. While the presence of a visitor, such as a volunteer, is important, all hospice personnel must be skilled in relating to the dying person and bridging the gap of isolation through meaningful relationships. The visitor needs to be able to relate comfortably with the dying person, communicating comfort and ease, dealing with silence and withdrawal on the part of the dying person, and to do all of these without expecting expressed appreciation.

In some ways visiting with the dying person can be the most significant responsibility for the hospice volunteer, whether the service is provided at home or in a residential facility. The team of volunteers can be carefully scheduled "around the clock," becoming a bastion of caring within the hospice program. Because of difficulties inherent in the assignment of hours for sitting with the isolated dying person, volunteers must be helped to avoid having feelings of isolation transferred to them. Volunteers helping to prevent the isolation of the dying person will need strong hospice community support and appreciation of their contribution. Such support is sensitive to early signs of fatigue, depression, isolation, or other symptoms that signal the need for help on the part of individual volunteers.

## Family

The person who comes to hospice for care is in many ways an extension of other people, family, and friends. The pain and trauma experienced during the period of dying is extended into the lives of many others. Other lives are upset; others feel the pain and anguish; others suffer as a life ends; and others are confused and bewildered.

Interwoven into this network of feelings and concern is the uncertainty that results from being unable to influence a cure. Feelings of helplessness and despair are inevitable under these circumstances. Family members, as well as other caretakers, must be helped to appreciate the importance of caring and the ability to make a significant contribution when a cure cannot be anticipated.

**Principle:** *The family together with the patient is the unit of care. Care directed toward the patient must include concern for other persons in his life who are important to him.*

**Discussion:** Hospice care is predicated upon an understanding of the intimate interrelationships, dependencies, and supports in the family relationships and the need to consider the total family as the client involved in hospice care. For purposes of this discussion, family is defined to include close personal associations, whether or not there are attachments of kinship and without judging whether there is positive or negative regard. The intermixing of close feelings, the sense of importance and of concern makes the individual part of the family relationship. In a sense, community or circle of significant others is what is meant by family.

Hospice care recognizes that the way every member of the family deals with the dying of one of its community influences the way that person will die and the ability of hospice to have impact on that death. In many cultures this will include extended family and clan or group. It will not be unusual to have as many as twenty people who are involved intimately with the patient and who will wish to be in the area where their loved one is dying. Families so defined must from the outset be involved in the care of the dying person and be considered along with the patient in the caring process.

Where children are part of the family constellation, they should be included in the hospice care both as part of the group involved in caring for someone who is dying and as recipients of services made available to all family members.

There is a unique relationship between children and the terminally ill that certainly must border on the spiritual. While the setting may trouble some children, others do not seem frightened in the presence of a dying person.

One day a six-year-old child visiting a relative in hospice wandered into the room of another resident. Later when he was found by a member of the staff the child was sitting quietly with his small hand in the hand of the elderly resident. Innocence and wisdom converged. Nothing was being said but each lovingly gazed at the other. When the child was questioned about the visit he merely responded, "She liked me and wanted me to stay; she's going to die, you know."

Rooms should be provided in the hospice inpatient unit where family members can sleep. A special kitchen/dining area should be provided so that families can dine together and bring home-prepared favorite meals to share with the family member. The hospice concept assumes that holidays are shared together. There are no restrictive visiting hours. Family members are welcome at any time, day or night. There are no age restrictions on visitors. Young children are welcomed instead of being restricted from maintaining close contacts with the dying person.

Family members are included in the planning of care and encouraged to continue to offer their own care in both the home care and inpatient aspects of the program. Hospice should at all times communicate that its intended role is to support the family in their caring rather than to take over. Decisions regarding the intensity of hospice staff involvement in the family care should be based on the readiness and capacity of the family to continue to provide care. Any hospice commitments to intensive care should be readily rescinded when the family is ready to undertake it. Transitory dependent family behavior should be understood and hospice should be ready to do more when the family needs more help.

A family's experiences connected with the death of one of its members will determine how surviving family members will deal with dying in the future. If hospice care clearly demonstrates that dying can occur without pain, with dignity, and with the dying person able to maintain contact and control, survivors are likely to develop more positive responses toward death and dying. The residual pain for family members will be reduced if they believe their loved one died an appropriate death. The bereavement will be easier because the extra trauma caused by witnessing the pain of dying will have been omitted, and family members will become advocates for humanizing care of the dying and thereby advocates of hospice programs.

At the outset of hospice care, each family member should be drawn into the most comfortable role possible for giving support to the dying person. The wishes of the family should be considered instructions for hospice staff. Obviously there will be situations where the family is in apparent conflict with the dying person. While priority must be shown for the dying person's interests, the skill of hospice staff should be used to reconcile or minimize differences in order to avoid conflicting pulls on the patient, family, or staff.

Unfortunately, there will be times when family conflict will interfere with the comfort of the patient, and hospice staff will have to advocate on behalf of the patient, sometimes restricting family involvement. This is especially true when the patient asks staff to intervene with family to establish limits on visiting hours, frequency of visits, or in assuming responsibility on behalf of the patient.

One hospice resident belonged to a large and loving family. When she was admitted to hospice she was very weak and fragile. Although she loved her family very much, their frequent visits in large numbers left her drained for hours. One day she asked a staff member to limit the numbers of persons and frequency of visits. She said she could not tell them because they would be hurt. She explained that she must not get so exhausted she could not "finish the things she had to do." At such a time staff must intervene to spare the resident the social obligations imposed by a well-meaning family.

While families in conflict may be reconciled at the time of a death, the focus of care must be on the person who is dying and not on the reconciliation. Hospice staff members may find dealing with continuing family conflict at the time of dying, with all of its distractions, one of the most demanding and disturbing parts of hospice care. It should be remembered that neither hospice care nor death itself may be able to change family behavior which staff may perceive to be inappropriate.

## Death of a Child

The death of a child is especially difficult for most people. Children are not supposed to die; therefore the death of children most particularly represents failure to the health care system.

Both family and health care providers are profoundly affected by a child's terminal illness, and all need support. The greatest supports offered at this time are those arising from the strength the family displays by providing care and comfort to the dying child. Health care providers gain support and reaffirmation of their roles by encouraging and guiding the family during the crisis.

The "role of hospice" should be in support of the family, providing back-up services when needed and teaching family members those skills needed to make the child comfortable.

The child needs the close personal care of family, and this care is usually not possible in a hospital, where staff assumes primary responsibility for care (Scipien, et al., 1975). Hospitalization may be traumatic to the child because it forces separation from family and the familiar and secure environment of home. Martinson (1976) suggests that when the family provides care in the home, the child and family find greater peace and comfort.

Siblings, grandparents, and friends can all be part of the caring team at home and can give the parents respite. Pets can also provide a source of comfort.

**Principle:** *Home care of a dying child is part of the care offered in hospice, with the parents as primary caregivers with support provided by the interdisciplinary hospice team.*

**Discussion:** The assumption that the hospital is the appropriate place for a child to die needs to be challenged. The role of the hospital is supported, for example, by current nursing textbooks in pediatric care where the nurse is taught the hospital is the care provider, the nurse the major caretaker, and family is encouraged to join in providing care (Marlow, 1977; Scipien, et al., 1975). In this approach, parents are helped by the support of nursing staff and parents are encouraged to give as much care as possible, while the nurse remains the primary caregiver.

The inappropriateness of children's dying in hospitals is made more understandable by the expectation that if any cure is possible, it will occur within the hospital setting. The hospital, with all its technology, represents the major hope for the prolongation of life. Home care for the child can be effective when parents and physician accept that cure-oriented treatment is no longer suitable.

The appropriateness of home care for the dying child has been advocated by Martinson and associates (1976) at the University of Minnesota School of Nursing. They list six criteria for determining when it is best for the child to remain at home with the parents as primary caregivers. Home care is appropriate when:

1. Cure-oriented treatment has been discontinued.
2. The child wants to be at home.
3. The parents want to have the child at home.
4. The parents recognize their ability to care for their ill child.
5. The nurse is willing to be an on-call consultant.
6. The child's physician is willing to be an on-call consultant.

The major thrust of home care under these circumstances is essentially an educational supportive experience for the caregiver, with teaching and counseling provided by the hospice team. Parents will need instruction in care procedures as well as recognition of possible changes in health status.

Hospice can teach parents how to provide comfort measures, how to suction, administer oxygen if needed, and give injections, if appropriate. The nurse can provide anticipatory guidance by outlining the possible complications that may arise. Martinson (1976) found that explaining what might happen helped parents by dispelling uncertainty, which was more frightening than understanding the situation. Caring for their dying child places the parents in control. The hospice home-care team can make sure that parents remain in control by giving them information, encouraging them by coaching, praising their efforts, and reassuring them that the care they are giving is good. When they understand the complications that may occur, parents can prepare for needed equipment or move the child to another location in the house if appropriate.

The problems that most commonly concern parents are hemorrhage, pain, seizures, and breathing difficulties. In Martinson's (1979) study, all these problems except pain occurred infrequently and could be anticipated.

Pain was of concern for most children dying at home. Oral drugs are preferable to injections as long as vomiting is not a problem. It was found that oral methadone combined with a tranquilizer (hydroxyzine) was effective (Martinson, 1977).

The rewards to the family of home care are very significant. Family members find they are more capable than they had expected, and there subsequently seems to be less family breakup than in other families that have suffered the loss of a child.

The role of hospice in the care of a child at home can be either as consultant and backup to the professional caregivers and provider of support for the parents, or as primary care provider. Depending on the situation, the hospice team can also provide direct bereavement services or act as consultant to others providing bereavement care.

It is not the intent of a hospice program to supplant others functioning to help families, but rather to provide knowledge, experience, and care if needed.

The child whose illness has been diagnosed as cancer or leukemia is often referred to a large regional pediatric oncology unit for care and treatment. A prolonged period of treatment includes frequent hospitalizations, putting the child and family in close contact with supportive care providers. These new supportive relationships become extremely important to the family and provide a continuity in the hospitalizations.

One of the reasons children are hospitalized during the final phase of an illness is to link the family to support of these caretakers with whom a bond has been established. Unfortunately the present system does not support the hospital-based staff's ability to continue this caring relationship. This should be a goal for hospital units serving children with terminal illnesses and appears to be an area that lends itself to a new, close working relationship between the hospital pediatric unit and the hospice unit. A unit that is either part of the hospital or community based could initiate the hospice home support role early in the treatment of the terminally ill child so that the significant relationships in support of parents would have time to be established. In the hospice relationship, the entire multidisciplinary team would be available to assist parents and would be associated with a program committed to home care.

The following case illustration of an attempt to provide home care for a dying child by a hospital inpatient unit helps demonstrate the significant role for a hospice home-care unit.

Tim, age six, was dying of leukemia. The parents and older siblings provided the necessary care at home supported by a pediatric resident and a nurse. The family had become very close to one of the night nurses and they "selected" each other. The nurse made home visits often and gave Tim and his family much needed support. Early one evening the child's condition became much worse. The family could not reach the physician or the nurse. They called the inpatient hospital unit and were told to bring the child in. The child died en route to the hospital, and the family was met by their "special nurse" in the emergency room.

The goal of a hospice home-care unit would have been to help the family keep the child at home until death. The desperate search for unavailable caretakers and the trauma of death in the automobile are problems a hospice care program would help overcome.

The preliminary work of Martinson and her associates in this area supports the idea that parents can provide care in their own home for a dying child. The program can be nurse-directed with the physician and other members of the hospice team serving as consultants to the parents.

The goal of such an effort is to enable the family to be the primary caregivers and to keep the child at home when this is the wish of the family. Obviously this should not preclude the use of an inpatient facility when this is the best way to provide care or when the family requests this level of support. Nor would we want to reduce the hope for recovery or remission that might be inherent in a hospital environment. Hospice care should provide the important option of support to families caring for a dying child at home. It is this latter option that is not presently available because of limits of financing home care, the unavailability of appropriate home-care supports, or because our prevailing attitudes have not been supportive of the feasibility of home care. Hospice should help dispel the myth that the hospital is the only appropriate place for children with terminal illness to die.

## Summary

The backdrop for developing a hospice care program must appropriately be set around concern for the individual for whom the care is oriented. Unquestionably, this should be the concern of all health care, but organizational demands, pressures of time, and distractions in purpose often have displaced the importance of the individual.

Hospice refocuses on the person needing care and recognizes that the uniqueness of each individual must be served to allow that person a death that is congruent with his or her lifestyle.

Hospice also recognizes that when a person is dying all who are close to that person experience the dual pains of shared suffering and of anticipated loss. The entire family should be considered the patient unit and, as such, be provided care as needed.

Before developing a hospice program, the following principles of hospice care should be understood and incorporated as the underlying precepts of hospice care:

- · Death with dignity.
- · Palliative care.
- · Individual control over life.
- · Significance of time.
- · Elimination of isolation.
- · Importance of the family.
- · Caring for children.

The application of these principles plus the control of pain and other distressing symptoms are basic to the philosophy of the hospice program.

# 3

## Control of Symptoms

Betty Koff

*The cornerstone of successful care of the chronically ill
patient is good pain control. It is impossible to give good
patient care, to manage the patient easily and well,
unless the patient has adequate pain control.*
> William M. Lamers, Jr.

*Before all else, palliative care must mean excellent
symptom control, eschewed by a health care team skilled
in clinical pharmacology.*

> Balfour M. Mount

SYMPTOM CONTROL, while often synonymous with the control of pain, should be viewed from a perspective of multiple sources of multiple symptoms. Pain may be exacerbated by social isolation or lack of control. Pain may be the product of physiological, psychological, spiritual, social, and emotional factors. An effective response to symptom control must therefore be based on a comprehensive multifaceted approach. Figure 3–1 shows the interrelationships of the multiple sources of pain and the components of an effective comprehensive response to symptom control.

Because providing control of symptoms is a major function of hospice, a planned, organized approach to understanding pain and controlling its symptoms is essential to any hospice program. Such an approach implies humane care, support, and concern based on knowledge of human behavior, response to illness, and physiological needs. If there were but one area in which hospice care could contribute to the well-being of terminally ill patients and their families, it would be to provide physical and emotional comfort.

Discomfort, pains of dying, misery, or whatever term is chosen to describe the host of problems and experiences of many dying persons, is not a simple or unidimensional situation of cause and effect. The distress being experienced may begin as a physiological entity, for example, nausea or pain that causes the person to change the way he feels about food or limits his ability to care for himself, or move about. These limitations will alter his lifestyle and probably will profoundly affect his feelings about himself, his family, and his very existence. The symptoms experienced frequently confirm fears that his condition is worse and heighten anxiety about having more pain and further discomfort. Pain, discomfort, and anguish are usually compounded of mental, physical, social, and spiritual elements. Because symptoms have many causes, alleviation of them must be multidimensional.

One example of such an approach is seen in a patient who had severe

*Editor's note:* This chapter, dealing with symptom control in some detail, may seem at first to be out of place in a general description of hospice care because it appears to be primarily directed to the nursing and medical staff. However, the control of pain and other disabling symptoms is a primary goal of hospice care, and if the hospice staff is to function as a multidisciplinary team, all hospice personnel should fully understand the approaches to symptom control.

We also believe that, when systematically organized and consistently practiced by the total staff, pain control can be realized for almost all hospice patients.

Betty Koff is a nurse-educator whose commitment to patient care has been the keystone of her career. Her material has been gathered through teaching, nursing practice, and extensive studies of hospice care.

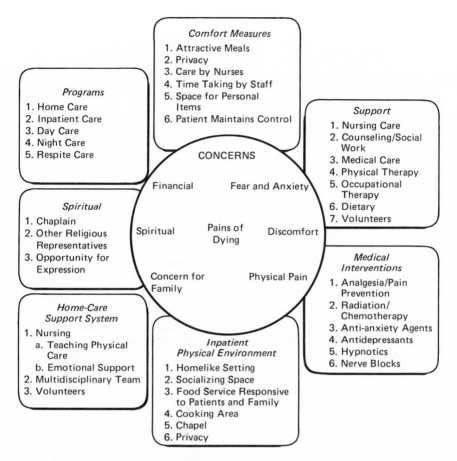

**Figure 3–1** Control of Symptoms

*Source:* Adapted from Dr. William Farr, Medical Director, Hillhaven Hospice, Tucson, Arizona.

back pain resulting from metastasis from breast cancer. Placed on a large dose of narcotic analgesic given regularly along with an antidepressant drug and a tranquilizer, she found her pain was partially controlled, but she was still tense and anxious. Suspecting that much of the pain was caused by anxiety, an attentive nurse discovered that the patient was afraid her tumor would spread to her face and cause severe disfigurement. After she had expressed her underlying fear, she was reassured that this would not happen. When her emotional concerns were quieted, the physical symptom control measures completely relieved her pain and she was able to function more normally (Lack, 1978).

It has become evident that relieving pain and discomfort is not only desirable, but is also achievable. The experiences of hospice programs in

Great Britain and in the United States have demonstrated the efficacy of symptom control. Saunders (1976) cites successful pain control in 98 percent of the cases at St. Christopher's Hospice.

The knowledge needed to control distressing symptoms is available. It takes commitment and determination to make such control available to terminally ill patients. It may be necessary to overcome prejudices such as those rejecting the use of narcotic analgesics in patients who have a short time to live. Most physicians and nurses in practice today have learned that narcotic analgesics can cause addiction and that increasing doses are needed in order to achieve the effect desired. Studies by Twycross (1975) and Mount (1976) in the use of narcotic analgesics (heroin and morphine) for chronic, severe pain do not support these concerns about addiction or tolerance to the drugs. Vere (1978) tends to blame physicians who prescribe drugs p.r.n. (as required), which inevitably leads to inadequate pain control. "If pain had not become uncontrolled, why would the next dose be 'required'?" Frequently physicians stop short of using a dose sufficient to control pain, and nurses are reluctant to administer narcotics on a regular basis (Valentine et al., 1978). The only truly effective way to relieve chronic, severe pain has been found to be through the use of narcotic analgesics administered regularly. This kind of regimen makes it possible to deal with other distressing symptoms by providing good care.

**Principle:**    *Care in a hospice program is directed toward overcoming pain and suffering by controlling the symptoms that cause or promote distress.*

**Discussion:**    It is important to understand the problem of pain as experienced by terminally ill persons.

Pain is frequently associated with illness, particularly when cancer is the diagnosis. However, only about 50 percent of persons with cancer experience pain and 10 percent of these have only mild pain. Of the remaining 40 percent, approximately half will need help in dealing with the symptom (Twycross, 1975).

Usually pain is a useful symptom, signaling that something is wrong; pain is useful in uncovering a problem. For example, abdominal pain of a certain duration and intensity may be a symptom of an inflamed appendix. Pain causes the sufferer to consult a physician, who may then diagnose the problem and treat it successfully.

Pain can be characterized as being acute, such as that experienced in the case of trauma or appendicitis, or chronic, which describes pain that persists over a long period of time—weeks or months. Pain is also described from the standpoint of intensity as mild, moderate, or severe. Acute pain can usually be endured because the underlying cause is usually known and its duration is relatively short, as in the cases of pain after surgery or resulting from injury (Valentine et al., 1978).

Chronic pain, if severe, is usually harder to bear. Its very persistence tends to dominate the life of the person experiencing it, interfering with every movement, including eating and sleeping. It frequently leaves the individual feeling anxious and isolated from others because he alone *feels* the pain (Valentine et al., 1978; Saunders, 1978). Dying with chronic unrelenting pain is one of the greatest fears of the terminally ill cancer patient (Farr, 1978).

In some situations severe, continuous pain defies verbal description. In a series of pictures painted by patients at St. Christopher's Hospice there were vivid illustrations of being totally isolated from the world by the encircling "muscles of tension," sudden jabs of pain on movement, and the feeling of being impaled on a red-hot iron (Saunders, 1978).

A word about pain perception is in order. Pain is a subjective symptom that is felt only by the individual experiencing it. Pain perception is not merely a function of the amount of physical injury or damage to tissues or organs, but also is determined by the level of anxiety, expectations of the onslaught of pain, the individual's personality, past experience with illness and pain, fear of disfigurement, fear of impending death, and worries about financial or family matters (Saunders, 1976).

While the person experiencing severe constant pain perceives it firsthand, family members and others involved with the individual's life feel sympathetic discomfort and may feel helpless to give comfort. Many family members suffer traumatic memories of the pain experienced by their loved ones long after the death of that individual. Parkes (1977), as social psychiatrist at St. Christopher's Hospice, interviewed more than 200 persons whose spouses had died of cancer one year earlier. He found that unrelenting pain was the symptom most vividly remembered. What the family members described as "pain" after a year had elapsed was not only physical suffering; they included social, psychological, and spiritual aspects.

Pain, or the fear of pain, is an all-encompassing feeling, imprisoning the person who experiences it and preventing his thinking or feeling any other sensation. Being freed from pain, or the fear of having pain, makes a person feel safe, and this feeling of safety gives him independence to be and to live. Relieving pain and preventing pain prolongs living and permits the individual to experience other thoughts and sensations. Providing temporary relief of pain is inadequate because the person knows his awful visitor will return, and he anticipates the oncoming sensation with dread. Then, as soon as pain does return, the skeletal muscles become tense, intensifying the sensation of pain and its torment. The world for that individual is "all pain" (Saunders, 1976).

Because many factors are involved in pain perception, a successful approach to pain relief requires both knowledge and analysis of all the elements involved in the patient's situation as well as information regarding available methods for relieving pain. Analysis of the patient's situation requires the following:

- Thorough assessment of the patient's complaints.
- Awareness of physical, emotional, and social components.
- Knowledge of patient's disease state.
- Information regarding family and financial matters.

## Assessment

The first step in giving care is the assessment of the patient's status. One question can be asked; that is, how is the patient "being" in spite of physical deterioration? What are the problems the patient perceives in order of importance to him? The priority in meeting needs may be dependent upon the *degree* to which there is interference with physical functioning.

Assessment requires that the patient be heard through verbal statements, body language, gestures, and voice tones. All these forms of communication are important to the message the patient sends to his caregivers and others. It takes a skilled and perceptive listener to pick up important clues. The nurse and others must be available to listen. Nurses frequently ask patients, "How are you today?" That question can be asked in the most casually offhand manner, which signals the patient that a casual, meaningless answer is in order. The same question asked in a tone of voice which implies real concern, with body language that gives the same message of concern, can be the beginning of information gathering if the nurse waits, observes, and takes the time to hear the real complaints and concerns of the patient and/or family member. Listening, then, is an important tool for the person assessing the needs of the dying patient.

A thorough assessment of the patient's responses will enable the caregiver to observe the patient's emotional state to learn, for example, whether the individual is depressed or anxious. Depression and anxiety lower the individual's threshold to perceive pain and may actually increase the need for a pain-relieving drug (analgesic). Treating the anxiety or depression by giving information or through the use of counseling and/or drugs can do much to reduce the amount of analgesic drugs or make the dosage given more effective (Shanfield and Killingworth, 1977).

The meaning that pain has for an individual and the way that person deals with pain are influenced by his cultural background. Past experience with pain, emotional factors, environment and expectations may prescribe the way an individual behaves in response to pain. In some cultures pain may be seen and accepted as part of the human condition. In others, pain may be viewed as part of the human condition, but not accepted as such. In some cultures stoicism and emotional control may be highly regarded; in others people may be expected to react emotionally when in pain. In the United States, pain tends not to be accepted, and measures are instituted to control or eliminate it. The prevailing cultural belief system tends to influence both what individuals do about pain and what they expect from caregivers who might help them relieve pain (Benoliel and Crowley, 1974).

A study by Davitz, Sameshina and Davitz (1976) indicates that nurses of different cultures respond in various ways to their patients' perception of pain and suffering. For example, Japanese people value control of feelings so that pain or suffering may not be openly expressed. Japanese nurses tended to infer that their Japanese patients suffered a high degree of physical pain and psychological discomfort. American nurses, in contrast, assumed that Oriental patients felt far less pain than patients of other ethnic backgrounds. American nurses probably assumed a greater congruence between behavior and experience than did Japanese nurses. Native Americans, like Orientals, tend to suppress strong feelings and may suffer silently. The non-Indian nurse can be misled into believing the patient is not having much discomfort. As a result, the pain and discomfort may not be relieved.

Another factor that influences pain perception is stress. Pain is increased with increased stress. Some sources of stress relate to family conflicts and financial problems. Many patients with a long-term illness find themselves financially depleted near the end of life. Some may feel that they have not provided sufficiently for their survivors and may experience guilt feelings as a result. If the patient has a family with young children, the stress and anxiety for that patient may be heightened, requiring interpersonal supports from members of the care team. In summary, it may be said that care of the total patient and family with knowledge of all the influences involved, and not merely treatment of a symptom, is the approach needed.

Dying patients not only have needs for pain relief and measures that prevent pain, but also needs for comfort and safety. The goal of care is to promote and maintain physiological functioning for as long as possible. Physiological needs are the foundation of a person as a physical being and therefore take precedence over needs such as the social or emotional. Once physiological needs are met, the person can deal with other aspects of his life. Some common problems that interfere with physiological functioning, especially in people with cancer, are pain, loss of appetite, nausea, vomiting, constipation, diarrhea, shortness of breath, immobility, incontinence, and skin breakdown.

A study by McKorkle and Young (1978) identified the following

**Table 3–1**   Guide for Pain Assessment

---

1. Location (anatomical site)
2. Description (aching, sharp, knife-like)
3. Intensity (mild, moderate, severe)
4. Duration (constant, intermittent)
5. Response to Pain (crying, immobility, withdrawal)
6. Current Relief Measures (what helps? what makes pain worse?)

---

symptoms as listed by terminally ill cancer patients to be the most distressing: nausea, mood changes, decreased appetite, insomnia, pain, limitations in mobility, fatigue, change in bowel function, difficulty concentrating, and change in appearance.

Assessment of the patient's physical complaints may be expedited by the use of data-collecting tools which some authors (Melzack et al., 1976; Twycross, 1976) have developed. Some use a chart of the body with a figure drawing on which is recorded a description of the pain as well as a mark locating the area where it occurs and the adjective which best describes the feeling. Such informational tools can frequently pinpoint an underlying problem; it cannot be assumed that pain is always caused by the malignant process of cancer. Constipation, fecal impaction, ulcers in the gastro-intestinal tract, bedsores, and muscle spasm may be responsible, and all these can be ameliorated by specific treatment. For this reason, it is wise to have several members of the care team assess the patient carefully to determine his disease state.

Usually it is a professional nurse or physician who collects this type of information, but other staff should also be involved.

Several tools are available for pain and for symptom assessment. It is suggested that hospice staff select such an assessment to assure that each patient problem is accurately defined so the most successful response to pain control can be determined. Among assessment methods that have been developed are the six described in Table 3–1.

The "Guide for Pain Assessment" can be used by nursing staff members as a data-collecting tool in their assessment of the quality, quantity, location, and responses to pain.

McGill-Melzack Pain Questionnaire

The McGill-Melzack Pain Questionnaire is a more detailed data-collecting tool originally developed to study the effectiveness of Brompton's mixture (explained later in greater detail) and to compare the results from its use with those from other more traditional methods of pain control. This questionnaire (Figure 3–2) could be used as it stands or adapted for use in a hospice program.

Patient's Name _____ Date _____ Time _____ am/pm

Analgesic(s) _____ Dosage _____ Time Given _____ am/pm

_____ Dosage _____ Time Given _____ am/pm

Analgesic Time Difference (Hours):    +4    +1    +2    +3

PRI: S _____ A _____ E _____ M(S) ____ M(AE) ____ M(T) ____ PRI(T) ____
      (1-10)   (11-15)   (16)    (17-19)    (20)      (17-20)    (1-20)

| 1. FLICKERING ____ | 11. TIRING ____ | PPI ____ COMMENTS: |
| QUIVERING ____ | EXHAUSTING ____ | |
| PULSING ____ | | |
| THROBBING ____ | 12. SICKENING ____ | |
| BEATING ____ | SUFFOCATING ____ | |
| POUNDING ____ | | |
| | 13. FEARFUL ____ | |
| 2. JUMPING ____ | FRIGHTFUL ____ | |
| FLASHING ____ | TERRIFYING ____ | |
| SHOOTING ____ | | |
| | 14. PUNISHING ____ | |
| 3. PRICKING ____ | GRUELLING ____ | |
| BORING ____ | CRUEL ____ | |
| DRILLING ____ | VICIOUS ____ | |
| STABBING ____ | KILLING ____ | |
| LANCINATING ____ | | |
| | 15. WRETCHED ____ | |
| 4. SHARP ____ | BLINDING ____ | |
| CUTTING ____ | | |
| LACERATING ____ | 16. ANNOYING ____ | |
| | TROUBLESOME ____ | |
| 5. PINCHING ____ | MISERABLE ____ | |
| PRESSING ____ | INTENSE ____ | |
| GNAWING ____ | UNBEARABLE ____ | |

| 5. CRAMPING ____ | 17. SPREADING ____ | ACCOMPANYING | SLEEP: |
| CRUSHING ____ | RADIATING ____ | SYMPTOMS: | GOOD ____ |
| | PENETRATING ____ | NAUSEA ____ | FITFUL ____ |
| 6. TUGGING ____ | PIERCING ____ | HEADACHE ____ | CAN'T SLEEP ____ |
| PULLING ____ | | DIZZINESS ____ | |
| WRENCHING ____ | 18. TIGHT ____ | DROWSINESS ____ | COMMENTS: |
| | NUMB ____ | CONSTIPATION ____ | |
| 7. HOT ____ | DRAWING ____ | DIARRHEA ____ | |
| BURNING ____ | SQUEEZING ____ | | |
| SCALDING ____ | TEARING ____ | COMMENTS: | FOOD INTAKE: |
| SEARING ____ | | | GOOD ____ |
| | 19. COOL ____ | | SOME ____ |
| 8. TINGLING ____ | COLD ____ | | LITTLE ____ |
| ITCHY ____ | FREEZING ____ | | NONE ____ |
| SMARTING ____ | | | |
| STINGING ____ | 20. NAGGING ____ | ACTIVITY: | COMMENTS: |
| | NAUSEATING ____ | GOOD ____ | |
| 9. DULL ____ | AGONIZING ____ | SOME ____ | |
| SORE ____ | DREADFUL ____ | LITTLE ____ | |
| HURTING ____ | TORTURING ____ | NONE ____ | |
| ACHING ____ | | | |
| HEAVY ____ | PPI 0 No Pain ____ | COMMENTS: | |
| | 1 Mild ____ | | |
| 10. TENDER ____ | 2 Discomforting ____ | | |
| TAUT ____ | 3 Distressing ____ | | |
| RASPING ____ | 4 Horrible ____ | | |
| SPLITTING ____ | 5 Excruciating ____ | | |

**Figure 3–2**  McGill-Melzack Pain Questionnaire

*Source:* Ronald Melzack, *C.M.A. Journal,* September 17, 1976. Reprinted with permission.

Using the McGill-Melzack Pain Questionnaire, adapted for study of effects of the Brompton mixture, descriptors fall into four major groups: sensory, 1 to 10; affective, 11 to 15; evaluative, 16; and miscellaneous, 17 to 20. The rank value for each descriptor is based on its position in the word set. The sum of the rank values is the "pain-rating index" (PRI). The "present pain intensity" (PPI) is based on a scale of 0 to 5.

### TWYCROSS BODY CHART

The body chart suggested for use by Twycross (1976) is useful in pinpointing the specific locus of pain. One of the problems this author has noted is the difficulty nurses and/or physicians experience when attempting to state where pain is located, especially if specific anatomical landmarks are not used. When terminology is not standardized, a drawing such as that shown in Figure 3–3 can be very helpful.

### ASSESSMENT OF PHYSIOLOGICAL AND EMOTIONAL FUNCTIONING

The assessment of physical functioning can be separated in a systematic progression of steps in order of their physiological importance, beginning with oxygen needs, which includes respiratory and circulatory components. The status of the patient's fluids and electrolytes is next in order of priority, followed by nutrition, elimination, activity and mobility, rest, and need for comfort. The order in which the needs are met or care is given is based upon the problems defined as a result of systematic assessment.

The assessment scale of physiological and emotional functioning shown in Table 3–2 is a sample of one method useful in strengthening observation technique and collecting significant data.

### SYMPTOMS OF CONCERN TO PATIENTS

A fourth tool for use in assessing problems experienced by terminally ill patients was developed from the list of symptoms that patients identified as causing them concern.

McKorkle and Young (1978) developed this symptom distress scale with ten items identified as symptoms that were of concern to patients. They included nausea, mood, appetite, insomnia, pain, mobility, fatigue, bowel pattern, concentration, and appearance. The tool was developed in order to control and manage the distress experienced by terminally ill cancer patients and others with terminal diseases (see Table 3–3).

Each symptom is rated on a scale of one to five. A score of one represents either no distress or minimum distress for a particular symptom. A

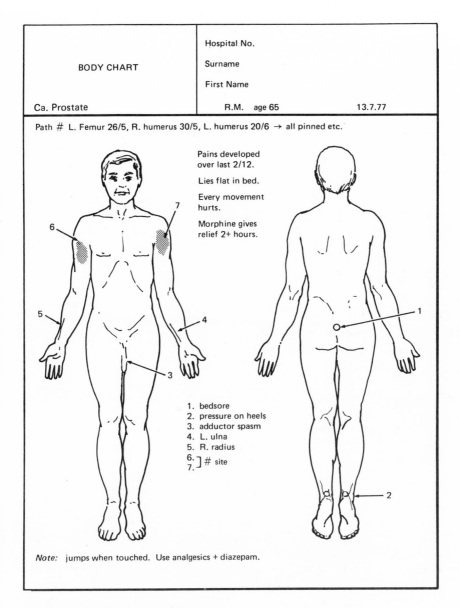

| BODY CHART | Hospital No. |
| | Surname |
| | First Name |
| Ca. Prostate | R.M.  age 65 |

13.7.77

Path # L. Femur 26/5, R. humerus 30/5, L. humerus 20/6 → all pinned etc.

Pains developed over last 2/12.

Lies flat in bed.

Every movement hurts.

Morphine gives relief 2+ hours.

1. bedsore
2. pressure on heels
3. adductor spasm
4. L. ulna
5. R. radius
6. ⎤ # site
7. ⎦

*Note:* jumps when touched. Use analgesics + diazepam.

**Figure 3–3**  Twycross Body Chart

*Source:* Reproduced from *Topics in Therapeutics*, volume 4, edited by D. W. Vere, by courtesy of Pitman Publishing Co., Tunbridge Wells, England.

**Table 3–2**    Assessment of Physiological and Emotional Functioning
Symptom Questionnaire

| Common Problem | Intensity Scale * | | | | | | Comments |
|---|---|---|---|---|---|---|---|
| | 0 | 1 | 2 | 3 | 4 | 5 | |
| 1. Pain | | | | | | | |
| 2. Short of breath, Dyspnea | | | | | | | |
| 3. Cough | | | | | | | |
| 4. Edema, Dehydration | | | | | | | |
| 5. Loss of Appetite | | | | | | | |
| 6. Nausea and Vomiting | | | | | | | |
| 7. Dysphagia | | | | | | | |
| 8. Constipation or Diarrhea | | | | | | | |
| 9. Incontinence    Bowel                        Bladder | | | | | | | |
| 10. Weakness, Difficulty Moving | | | | | | | |
| 11. Restlessness | | | | | | | |
| 12. Skin Breakdown | | | | | | | |
| 13. Anxiety/Depression | | | | | | | |
| 14. Disorientation (Time/Place/Person) | | | | | | | |
| 15. Other Problems Define: | | | | | | | |

\* Explanation of intensity scale:
  0   no symptoms present
  1   mild
  3   moderate
  5   severe

score of five represents extreme distress, with scores of two, three, and four representing intermediate levels of distress. The patient can be asked to place a circle around the number that most closely corresponds to his perceptions of distress.

Assessment of physiological needs is a continuous process because these needs are continually changing as the stage and degree of illness change. For example, in the case of an individual suffering from cancer affecting the large intestine, the immediate problem might be to relieve the pain and discomfort of cramps in the abdomen, and as the disease progresses, the abdomen may enlarge, pushing up on the diaphragm and interfering with respiration. This requires a reassessment to take the new problem into consideration.

**Table 3–3** Symptoms of Concern to Patients

| | | | | | | | |
|---|---|---|---|---|---|---|---|
| Nausea | I feel as sick as I could possibly be | 5 | 4 | 3 | 2 | 1 | I do not feel sick |
| Mood | Could not feel more miserable | 5 | 4 | 3 | 2 | 1 | Could not feel happier |
| Appetite | Can't face food at all | 5 | 4 | 3 | 2 | 1 | Normal appetite |
| Insomnia | Couldn't have been worse | 5 | 4 | 3 | 2 | 1 | A perfect night |
| Pain | Worst pain I've ever had | 5 | 4 | 3 | 2 | 1 | No pain |
| Mobility | Not able to get around | 5 | 4 | 3 | 2 | 1 | Able to do everything |
| Fatigue | Couldn't feel more tired | 5 | 4 | 3 | 2 | 1 | Am not tired at all |
| Bowel Pattern | The worst I've ever had | 5 | 4 | 3 | 2 | 1 | Normal bowel pattern |
| Concentration | Cannot concentrate at all | 5 | 4 | 3 | 2 | 1 | Normal concentration |
| Appearance | The worst I've ever had | 5 | 4 | 3 | 2 | 1 | Appearance has not changed |

*Source:* Ruth McKorkle and Katherine Young. "Development of a Symptom Distress Scale" (*Cancer Nursing,* vol. 1, no. 5, p. 375, October 1978). Copyright by Masson Publishing USA, Inc., New York.

The previous discussion has focused on assessment as a prerequisite to control of distressing symptoms. Once the problems are understood it is then possible to intervene appropriately to provide relief.

The usual notes of caution should be raised. Tools are only as good as the people using them. Use of the tools should not add to the patient's distress, and the tools are essentially useless unless they are only the first part of the process of relieving the distressing symptoms. That many can provide in-depth analysis without the use of any tool is not questioned nor should we overlook the need of some practitioners to increase their assessment skills. The ultimate judgment about any assessment tool is not in the assessment tool or its use, but rather in the successful reduction of pain and other distressing symptoms.

## Relief of Symptoms: Pain

There are many ways to relieve pain. Drugs are very useful and are perhaps the best known. Other methods of relieving pain are nursing and medically therapeutic measures that include: positioning for comfort, massage, heat, radiation therapy, chemotherapy, surgery, supportive activities, and counseling. For some patients there are surgical procedures to interrupt nerve pathways that conduct pain; this may produce total relief.

Radiation or chemotherapy given to reduce tumor size may produce pain relief (Twycross, 1975).

In cases where there is inflammation of the bone caused by a reaction to tumor growth, favorable response has been obtained through the use of anti-inflammatory drugs such as aspirin, indomethacin (Indocin), phenylbutazone (Butazoledin), and Prednisone. It should be pointed out that some of these drugs cause undesired side effects and Twycross (1975) favors aspirin instead of the other drugs for that reason. Aspirin is not only useful for its anti-inflammatory effect, but also for its analgesic effect and its wide margin of safety. However, patients with bleeding tendencies should avoid aspirin. Physical mobility should be maintained for as long as possible to prevent physical complications of immobility as well as the emotional and social aspects of being bedridden.

When other measures to relieve pain are not appropriate, additional analgesics are used, depending on the intensity of pain. Aspirin may be combined with codeine or Darvon (propoxyphene). Where there is severe intractable pain, the situation becomes more complex because drugs used to overcome it may have some undesirable side effects.

Methods of pain control and studies cited in this section are based on an adult population and do not include children. Table 3–4 presents an outline of the approaches suggested for the treatment of pain caused by advanced cancer.

Treating severe, intractible, and persistent pain usually requires the use of potent analgesic drugs. Some authors (Mount et al., 1976) have outlined as goals in such circumstances:

1. Clarifying the underlying cause of pain.
2. Preventing pain by anticipating its recurrence.
3. Erasing the memory of pain.
4. Keeping the patient alert.
5. Considering ease of administration.

*Clarifying the underlying cause of pain* can be accomplished after a thorough assessment of the patient's situation. As explained earlier, the pain may be the result of tumor growth, muscle spasm, bone or joint inflammation, constipation, bedsores (decubiti), or any number of other factors, such as depression, fear, anger, etc. The drug or program chosen to relieve pain will depend upon the cause of pain as well as its intensity.

*Preventing pain by anticipating its recurrence* implies giving a pain-relieving drug on a regular rather than "as needed" basis. Traditionally those experiencing pain wait until they feel pain before they take a drug to relieve it. They must first experience the feeling and then wait until the drug is absorbed into the bloodstream in order for relief to begin. The time it takes for a drug to work depends upon the route of administration and the integrity and efficiency of various organ systems of the body. In order to prevent incessant pain, the drug must be maintained at a certain level in the blood, so that the pain is no longer perceived. This blood level can only be maintained by regular administration around the clock; an additional dose of drug is given before the effect of the previous dose has worn off (Twycross, 1975).

*Erasing pain memory* can be achieved through regular administration of the pain-relieving drug before the patient experiences the return of pain. The anticipation of pain promotes increased anxiety and fear, which then heighten the perception of the pain. In order to erase the memory of pain, it is first necessary to prevent the pain from reoccurring (Twycross, 1975).

*Keeping the patient alert,* neither sedated nor euphoric, is a challenge because narcotic analgesics tend to promote drowsiness. Many patients find themselves trapped in the vicious cycle of pain interspersed with a drowsy state. When awake, the person is in misery, and when the pain is relieved he dozes. Several authors (Twycross, 1975; Mount et al., 1976; and Farr, 1978) report that morphine given orally at a level calculated to relieve pain depending upon its intensity does not cause drowsiness or confusion. If sedation is noted, it is usually transient or indicative of the advanced state of the disease, rather than the effect of the drug.

*Ease of administration* can be accomplished by oral administration of analgesics, which permits the person to maintain a degree of independence and mobility. Taking medications by mouth rather than injection makes it possible for many patients to remain at home. Oral administration of drugs does not require dispensing by a skilled person. Injection of substances several times during the day can be physically uncomfortable and lead to skin breakdown. Medication in the form of a liquid is easy for the debilitated patient to sip and easier to swallow than pills (Mount et al., 1976). Liquid medication also permits an ease in adjusting the dosage without the volume, thereby reducing the patient's anxiety at having to take larger pills or more frequent medication.

There are a number of preparations in use that prevent pain, erase the memory of pain, keep the patient alert, and are easy to administer. The best known among the drugs used is Brompton's mixture, developed by Brompton's Chest Hospital in England. The effectiveness of the mixture in relieving chronic severe pain was established at St. Christopher's Hospice. Originally, Brompton's mixture was a liquid containing heroin, cocaine, alcohol, and chloroform water in a flavoring syrup. In the United States and Canada, morphine has been substituted for heroin. As a result of experience, St. Christopher's Hospice made modifications; its staff now has substituted morphine for heroin because morphine was found to be effective, and has omitted cocaine, which was found to add to the undesirable side effects such as confusion (Twycross, 1976). Therefore, in

**Table 3–4** Treatment of Pain in Cancer

| Mechanism | Analgesic | Co-Analgesic | Nondrug Treatment | Other Measures |
|---|---|---|---|---|
| 1. Soft tissue infiltration | Severe pain MORPHINE CLASS | aspirin chemotherapy to reduce tumor | radiation therapy | 1. Careful positioning and movement, change positions if possible, heat if helpful |
| 2. Bone involvement | | | | 2. Careful positioning and movement, get out of bed if possible, protect area of involvement |
| 3. Nerve compression | Moderate pain CODEINE CLASS | prednisolone | nerve block | 3. Careful handling and movement, supportive activities |
| 4. Raised cerebral pressure | | dexamethasone | compression sleeve | 4. Elevate head of bed 10°–30°, quiet, cool room |
| 5. Lymphedema | | diuretic | | 5. Elevate part of body involved, assist with moving, gentle handling |

| | Drug treatment | Nerve block | Nursing/other measures |
|---|---|---|---|
| 6. Abdominal visceral | | | |
| a. epigastric | Mild pain ASPIRIN CLASS | coeliac axis | 6a. Heat if helpful, small attractive meals or liquids, supportive activities |
| b. hypogastric | | ganglion block *(presacral block) | 6b. If abdomen distends move carefully, assist with eructation |
| 7. Ulceration—infection | antibiotic | | 7. Protect ulcer, prevent further irritation and/or infection |
| 8. Constipation | | | 8. Check for fecal impaction, stool softeners, high-bulk diet if possible, enema |
| 9. Second pathological process | Specific treatment | | |

* Use of nerve blocks for lower abdominal pain limited by probability of causing urinary retention.

Source: Adapted from R. G. Twycross, "Bone Pain in Advanced Cancer," in Topics in Therapeutics, vol. 4, edited by D. W. Vere, by courtesy of Pitman Medical Publishing Co., Tunbridge Wells, England.

**Table 3–5**  Brompton's Mix for 1 qt. (1000 cc.)

| | |
|---|---|
| Morphine Sulfate | 150 mg. per 10 cc. |
| Cocaine | 100 mg. per 10 cc. |
| Ethyl Alcohol | 1.8 cc. per 10 cc. |
| Grenadine Syrup | 1.875 cc. per 10 cc. |
| Water q.s. to make 1000 cc. | |

| *Modified Brompton's Mix* | |
|---|---|
| Morphine Sulfate | 10 mg. per 5 cc. |
| * Grenadine Syrup | 1 part |
| Water | 4 parts |
| Water q.s. to dilute to morphine 5 mg. = 5 cc. | |

* May substitute cherry syrup. It is also suggested that the addition of a small amount of Parabens will control the occasional growth of fungus in the mixture.

*Source:* D. Jacobs, Regional Director, American Society of Consultant Pharmacists, Tucson, Arizona.

many hospices, the *modified* Brompton's mixture now includes only morphine sulfate and a flavoring such as grenadine syrup (Farr, 1978). References made to Brompton's mixture (or cocktail) may be to either of these variations, as there is not at present a single standardized formula.

The pharmacological formulae for Brompton's mix and modified Brompton's most commonly used are shown in Table 3–5.

Brompton's mixture in its original or modified form is easy to administer and swallow.

Groups in different parts of the United States are using still other solutions for pain control. Valentine, Steckel, and Weintraub (1978) tested an elixir containing methadone, ethyl alcohol (for its palatability) and flavoring. They called their preparation "Val-Steck" elixir. They found that 5 to 10 ml. (one to two teaspoons) of Val-Steck were preferable to four teaspoons of Brompton's in its standard dose in that the patient could take a smaller amount. They also found that mixing the methadone with an amphetamine offered the best pain relief. Their study sample was small and much more needs to be learned of the use of methadone for pain control. Because methadone is excreted slowly from the body, it has been noted that hospice patients repeatedly treated with it died more quickly than those given equivalent doses of morphine. Twycross recommends against its repeated use (Vere, 1978). Dr. Richard Lamerton, Medical Director of St. Joseph's Hospice in London, recommends against methadone for much the same reasons; both physicians' experience with methadone in actual practice is that it tends to shorten life (Lamerton, 1977; Twycross, 1976).

Administering narcotics has several disadvantages, some from the standpoint of those receiving the drugs and some encountered by staff members responsible for giving them. Persons receiving narcotic analgesics, which include morphine and methadone, may become sedated, especially when the drug is first introduced. Other symptoms such as nausea, vomiting, and constipation may be observed, especially when the dose is moderately high (20 mg. of morphine). Nausea can be prevented if another drug from the phenothiazine group is given in conjunction with the narcotic. The phenothiazines are tranquilizers as well as antinauseant drugs and work in conjunction with the narcotic analgesic, making its pain-relieving qualities even more effective. Therefore, in actual practice in various hospice programs (Lack, 1978; Mount et al., 1976; Twycross, 1975; Farr, 1978), a modified Brompton's mixture is given with prochlorperazine (Compazine) or other phenothiazines. Constipation is the most frequent side effect encountered, and Farr (1978) suggests that each patient receiving the morphine solution be carefully checked and given a stool softener plus an occasional enema, if needed, to maintain adequate bowel functioning.

Because individual responses to narcotic analgesics vary, there should be flexibility in the doses used and frequency of administration as is demonstrated in Table 3–6.

The problems encountered by staff in administering a narcotic anal-

**Table 3–6**   Protocol for Use of Modified Brompton's Mixture *

Mixture: Morphine Sulfate 2 mg./ml.

Morphine Oral to Parenteral Ratio: Varies from 2:1–6:1

Protocol Dosage Changes:
1. Physician selects a dose to be given regularly q4h.
2. If pain not controlled, nurse will automatically increase the morphine to a maximum of 10 mg. per dose to control pain and continue on a q4h schedule. If the patient requires an increase of more than 10 mg. per dose, she calls for a new order.
3. If patient's pain is controlled but he is drowsy, shows evidence of confusion attributable to one drug, or sleeps at long intervals, the next scheduled dose will be held until the patient clears or shows evidence of pain. Subsequent morphine doses are decreased by a maximum of 10 mg. per dose until pain is controlled without the above side effects.
4. If nighttime sleep is not interrupted by pain, the patient is not awakened for medication.
5. If patient is awakened by pain day or night or awakens in the morning in moderate pain, nurse begins q4h schedule during sleeping hours.

Schedule Variation:
1. Nurse may give next scheduled dose 60 minutes earlier than ordered if patient has reappearance of pain.
2. Nurse is allowed to give one additional unscheduled dose of 10 mg. of oral morphine per 24 hours without an order.

Antiemetics and Tranquilizers:
A liquid form of an antiemetic or tranquilizer can be added to the mixture when nausea or anxiety is a significant problem. (Compazine 5 mg. orally)

* Used at Hillhaven Hospice, Tucson, Arizona.

gesic on a regular schedule include the fear of addicting patients. No one should fear that patients receiving these drugs will become addicted because it has been found that *undertreatment* encourages psychological dependence (Twycross, 1975). Progressive tolerance and escalating dosage requirements are often given as reasons for delaying the use of narcotics for pain control. However, the assumption underlying the belief is false. Mount et al. (1976) determined that a need for higher narcotic dosage indicated a worsening in the person's condition and was not a symptom of addiction. Once pain relief and prevention are achieved, the dose of narcotic is not escalated but is frequently lowered (Valentine et al., 1978).

Whatever the prescribed medication, it is important to give the narcotic at regular intervals and only to withhold or postpone a dose if the person is sleeping or groggy. Dosage should be at such a level that the individual remains alert, neither overwhelmed with distress nor incapacitated by drugs. There appears to be little in the literature that reports on pain relief in children. Martinson (1977) in a study related to home care of terminally ill children cites the use of merperedine (Demerol) given by injection. She stated in a personal conversation with one of the authors that in her experience methadone by mouth was effective. Several authors (Farr, 1978; Twycross, 1976) believe that merperedine (Demerol) is not useful in relieving chronic, severe pain.

The principles of successful use of opiates are through the use of applied pharmacology. These drugs can be dangerous, but when used with understanding can bring about much needed relief in chronic, severe pain. The principles are summarized in Table 3–7.

Table 3–8 summarizes the drugs frequently used to control pain.

**Table 3–7** Pharmacology of Morphine Drugs

| | | Used in Terminal Care | |
| | Problem | Pharmacological Principles | Practice |
|---|---|---|---|
| 1. | Which drug for severe pain? | Efficacy, not potency matters. Morphine more effective than most other opiates. | Use Morphine. |
| 2. | Will individuals need different doses? | Individual variation in responses to be expected. | Start with small doses, work up quickly until pain is controlled. |
| 3. | How should doses be spaced? | a. Range of effective plasma concentration.<br>b. Shape of plasma time-concentration.<br>c. Cumulation.<br>d. Physiology of pain. | a. Either give 4–5 times daily or use sustained release formulation.<br>b. No p.r.n. or as needed basis. |

**Table 3–7** *continued*

| Problem | Used in Terminal Care | |
|---|---|---|
| | *Pharmacological Principles* | *Practice* |
| 4. Route of administration? | a. Shape of plasma time-concentration curve. Plasma level in toxic range more likely with intravenous administration. Oral administration slower to peak, drug remains in useful range.<br>b. Respiratory depression may occur in toxic range. | Give drug orally whenever possible. If not, give subcutaneously. |
| 5. Is Methadone an alternative? | Cumulation-plasma half-time much longer than morphine. Metabolism of Methadone varies with time over series of doses. Shorter survival time for patients receiving drug in hospice programs. | Avoid Methadone. |
| 6. Can drugs be mixed? | Single receptor mechanism. | No gains expected from mixing drugs. |
| 7. Will dose need to be increased progressively? | a. Fact of tolerance.<br>b. Nature of tolerance. | Dose may need to be increased to achieve pain control. |
| 8. Will dependence occur? | Nature of dependence in those who suffer pain. | Forget it, except when withdrawing drug, then taper dose. |
| 9. Will there be undesirable effects of drug? | a. Spectrum of opiate effects.<br>b. Physiological antagonism.<br>c. Potentiation. | a. Use mixtures with phenothiazines.<br>b. Anticipate constipation, use stool softeners. |
| 10. Are there ethical problems? | | Treat for what remains of life, not for death. Let death be normal part of life. |
| 11. Will solutions keep on shelf? | Facts about solubility and stability of drugs. | Solutions can be stored. |

*Source:* Reproduced from "Pharmacology of Morphine Drugs Used in Terminal Care" in *Topics in Therapeutics* vol. 4, edited by D. W. Vere, by courtesy of Medical Publishing Co., Tunbridge Wells, England.

**Table 3–8**    Drugs Frequently Used for Pain Control

| Symptom | |
| --- | --- |
| Bone Pain Inflammation | *Anti-Inflammatory* <br> • Aspirin (ASA) <br> • Phenylbutazone (Butazolidin) <br> • Hydrocortisone (Prednisone) |
| Mild to Moderate Pain | *Mild-Moderate Analgesic* <br> • Codeine combined with ASA or Acetominophen <br> • Oxycodone (Percodan, Percocet) <br>   • Percodan—ASA, Phenacetin, Caffeine <br>   • Percocet—Contains Acetominophen |
| Severe Pain | • Morphine Sulfate Mixture (Modified Brompton's Mix) |

## Relief of Symptoms: Other Distressing Problems

Observing, collecting data (assessing), then intervening appropriately and evaluating the patient's situation is a cyclical process in the control of symptoms for those suffering from terminal illness. For example, the respiratory rate, quality of respirations, skin color, and pulse rate are some of the observations made in order to assess oxygen needs. If the patient is pale and having a difficult time breathing, the nurse will intervene to meet the patient's needs for oxygen by being sure the airway is patent, suctioning secretions, raising the head of the bed to utilize the force of gravity to assist in diaphragmatic excursion and, if appropriate, giving oxygen at a rate ordered by the physician. She will then evaluate the situation to see if her interventions have relieved the problem. The secretions, which are often heard as the dying person reaches the last days or hours of life, can be mitigated through the use of Hyoscine given subcutaneously (Saunders, 1976).

The need for fluids is physiologically second in importance by virtue of the fact that human beings can live approximately four minutes without oxygen, one or two days without fluid, and some weeks without food. The nurse will observe the skin, mucous membranes, and the patient's fluid intake and urinary output to determine whether the need for fluids is being adequately met. Assessment of electrolytes may be made by laboratory tests as well as by observing cardiac rate, checking for patient complaints of muscle cramping, twitching, level of consciousness, confusion, etc. Nursing measures to overcome electrolyte loss such as giving specific fluids to correct potassium depletion can be instituted if appropriate. Nutritional needs can be assessed by observing the patient's appetite and by eliciting subjective symptoms such as complaints of nausea, lack of appetite, or bloated feeling. Nursing measures such as serving small attractive meals, determining the patient's preferences, ordering special treats, and making mealtime a social experience can help in improving appetite. Several drugs can be used as appetite stimulants; they are alcoholic beverages before or with a meal and corticosteroids such as Prednisone in small doses, promoting a sense of well-being and improving appetite (Baines, n.d.).

Some patients are unable to eat or drink because they experience sore areas in the mucous membrane of the mouth. The excoriations and tenderness may be the side effects of chemotherapy. Whatever the cause, care should be taken to reduce irritation and offer foods which are neither acid nor alkaline. Fluids such as milk, egg nogs, etc. may be helpful, as well as high protein drinks. It may not be possible for the patient to chew, therefore soft foods such as custard, cottage cheese, applesauce, and mashed potatoes may be offered. The use of toothbrushes and glycerine or lemon swabs should be avoided. Mild saline solutions or commercial "toothettes" may be used for cleansing the mouth.

There are a number of drugs used to control nausea which can be given orally, rectally, or by injection. Among these are drugs mentioned earlier, phenothiazines such as Compazine, Phenergan, and Torecan. The route of administration should depend on the patient's condition as well as his wishes. Nausea and vomiting due to intestinal obstruction can often be controlled in the terminal phase of cancer by the use of adequate analgesics and antiemetics. Lomotil may be used to control painful cramping (Baines, n.d.).

Elimination needs can be easily assessed by eliciting information from the patient, observing bowel function, checking for impactions manually and by palpation and auscultation of the abdomen for bowel sounds and distention. As stated earlier, narcotic analgesics cause constipation, therefore a stool softener should be given daily to prevent the problem, and an occasional enema may be needed (Farr, 1978). Dietary addition of bran, sufficient fluids, and dried fruit (raisins, prunes, etc.) are also useful in promoting bowel elimination.

Loss of bowel and/or bladder control is usually very distressing to the patient as well as his family. Toileting the patient at frequent intervals, using an external catheter for men or an in-dwelling catheter may help. Prompt and meticulous skin care is required in the event of incontinence to prevent skin breakdown. Retention of urine can be assessed by checking the urinary output and by palpating the pelvic region of the abdomen for distention. Measures to relieve the retention, such as the use of catheters, can then be instituted.

Movement and activity are important not only psychologically, but also physiologically. Muscles that lie unused soon atrophy, and when an individual wants to move about he is unable to get the muscles to respond because they are weak. Ability to move is easily assessed by observing activity. If the patient is bedridden, the nurse can perform either an active or a passive range of joint motion exercises several times a day. If at all possible, bedridden patients should be transferred from bed to chair. Aids to ambulation, such as walkers, canes, and staff assistance, can also be used. The goal is to keep patients up and moving, using their muscles and avoiding immobility. Keeping active helps patients to rest and sleep better.

Assessing the need for hygiene and skin care means observing the condition of the skin for pressure areas, redness, skin breakdown, and state of hydration. Many terminally ill persons may be very thin, with little subcutaneous fat, while others may appear obese due to excess tissue fluid (edema). In either situation, skin breakdown is a potential problem. Many aids exist to prevent or ameliorate the problem; these include sheepskin pads, alternate pressure mattresses, "Gel" pads, and mattresses and water beds. Water beds can be made by purchasing a good quality air mattress, filling it halfway with water, and placing it on a standard mattress. This has the advantages of being lighter in weight than the standard water mattress, can be used in the home, and is far less expensive. When appropriate, the use of physical aids, changing position, gentle massage, skin lotions, or gentle heat will help increase comfort and prevent skin breakdown.

While the focus of this chapter has been on the control of pain and other physiological symptoms, it is important to note that disease and the treatment of disease may often cause bodily disfigurement. Such bodily changes may result in an alteration of body image, self-concept, and physical function. For example, chemotherapy frequently causes hair loss, and tumors that involve the liver usually cause significant weight loss, a puffy appearance due to fluid retention, and jaundice. Problems with bodily images may complicate efforts at pain reduction and need prompt and sensitive responses. Patients may be helped through the use of a wig, appropriate clothing, makeup, or other supportive efforts. Hospice's staff can play an important role by providing thoughtful demonstrations of caring when these side effects occur.

## Summary

Hospices have reason to be proud of their primary expertise in the ability to control pain and other symptoms. The 98 percent success rate in controlling pain reported in some hospice programs (Saunders, 1976) is an astonishing accomplishment and should earn for them a well-deserved reputation for providing outstanding pain control programs. This is a goal all hospice programs should aspire to reach.

Beyond that, it should be the goal of every hospice program to reach the 100 percent success rate in pain control, or to have the capacity to give every person using hospice services individual care that is most responsive to that person's need for pain and other symptom control. Satisfaction with anything less reflects a complacency that has no place in hospice care.

# 4

## The Program

**A Two-Edged Scythe**

*Is death kinder when it*
  *swoops down*
  *guts*
  *wrenches out the light?*
*Or when it is delivered subtly*
  *in small bleak bundles*
  *stamped with Medicare*
  *sealed with a 15% discount for Senior Citizens,*
*And in a wide assortment of little deaths*
  *no more salt*
  *no more sugar*
  *a plastic hip socket*
  *an eroded driver's license*
  *wavering memory*
  *crystal goblets that gather dust?*
*It is a moot question—*
*not mine to answer.*
*Something or somebody else*
*mulls the options.*

                    Helen C. Stark


*Moment to moment my heart did cry*
  *the ache so deep in our knowing*
*And now moment to moment that heart*
  *lessens, with so much togetherness and*
  *understanding.*

                    Daughter of a hospice patient

IN THE FRAMEWORK of hospice programs, the person served determines the program and should be the focal point of planning. This requires that the program be flexible and responsive to the patient's changing needs. In some ways, a hospice program evolves into a miniature health and social service system for the care of the dying.

Hospice care actually is dependent upon having available a complete balance among the several levels of care which together form the hospice continuum. Care for the dying at times may be offered in a hospice building; an inpatient program is essential to the full scope of hospice services enabling the continuity of levels of care, but many individuals will use hospice and not use the building itself.

Hospice is a concept—not a building. Hospice is a special program of caring that can be offered where it is needed.

> What people need most when they are dying is relief from the distressing symptoms of their disease, the security of a caring environment, sustained expert care, and the assurance they and their families won't be abandoned.
>
> The program of care that is tailored to meet each patient's special needs and blends the skill of physicians, nurses, social workers, pharmacists, psychiatrists, and clergy in an interdisciplinary team which also uses the talents of nonprofessionals and volunteers does much to ease the suffering of those who face death. (Craven and Wald, 1975)

Hospice is the community of caring people—staff, volunteers, family and friends—responding to an individual who, freed from the trauma of pain, is able to sustain an ongoing lifestyle.

The hospice program can be a variety of services, activities, and interventions offered by staff to fulfill the initial obligation of hospice: to control pain and other symptoms. Figure 4–1 shows an overview of hospice program goals.

## Support of Individual Lifestyle

Hospice stresses the continuation of living during the process of dying. Obviously life cannot be conducted "as usual" because the ravages of the disease process may preclude that option. But, however the person may change in response to changing body functioning, he remains an individual.

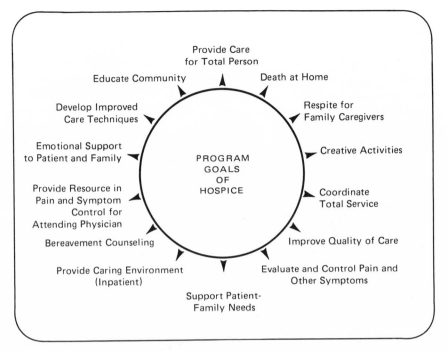

**Figure 4–1**  Hospice Program Goals

*Source:* Adapted from Dr. William Farr, Medical Director, Hillhaven Hospice, Tucson, Arizona.

**Principle:**  *Individual lifestyle should be supported as long as possible. Respect for the individual's ethnicity, cultural orientation, social and sexual preferences must be reflected in the services and program of hospice care.*

**Discussion:**  Opportunities to participate in creative activities may open new lifestyles or new ways of dealing with life's problems. For example, the outgoing, extroverted individual may appreciate opportunities for socialization in the hospice environment. Others may find new ways to express their personality or feelings about their life or may prefer to be alone. Whatever the individual's choice for socialization, hospice staff should support it.

Reminiscing sessions, creative writing, or poetry writing provide opportunities for communicating feelings, for verbalizing legacies, or for summarizing a life and its meaning. "Happy hours," birthdays, and holiday celebrations also offer opportunities to support an individual lifestyle.

Hospice programming, in spite of its orientation to respond to the problems of dying, serves living persons and should be activity-focused and future-oriented. These multiple goals are not mutually exclusive. It is inherent in the hospice philosophy that there is hope and future and that life should continue until death.

Hospice staff members must be cognizant of their own feelings regarding ethnic groups or sexual preferences when a patient's orientation differs from their own. The focus of the organized program should be to help individuals and families interact with others and support their needs for companionship. This requires a nonjudgmental attitude on the part of staff members.

The activities and orientation mentioned here are not limited to an inpatient program and can equally well be carried out in a home-care program. While individual lifestyle is more reasonably attainable within one's own household, people can become enslaved by illness and household responsibilities and be in need of a supporting hand to continue to live. Hospice staff members can help by providing a range of program opportunities to the individual at home.

SUPPORTING INDIVIDUAL LIFESTYLE THROUGH THE
SPIRITUAL DIMENSION*

To accept the hospice concept is to acknowledge that death is a normal phase in the life cycle. It is then inappropriate to support the notion of Camus that the worst thing in life is death—that life must be preserved at all costs and in all circumstances.

In earlier times every member of the family made a significant contribution to the total needs of the terminally ill in the home. Today the nuclear family is often fragmented by divorce or other kinds of separation, and the extended family is often separated by hundreds of miles. Today the most logical answer to the problem of caring for the terminally ill is the hospice.

The person who is soon to die mourns his impending loss. He must not be cheated of the opportunity to deal with what is happening to him. A climate of loving acceptance will enable him to respond to the meaning of his loss.

The goals of hospice care are to meet the total needs of the terminally ill, that is, physical, psychoemotional, and spiritual. While the physical needs of a person so diagnosed may be relatively easily satisfied, meeting

* Sister Teresa M. McIntier, CSJ, was invited to write the following section dealing with the spiritual dimension of hospice care because of her deep understanding of the multiple needs of hospice patients. She is both a nun and a registered nurse who holds a master's degree in nursing from the University of Arizona. By training and experience, she is accustomed to providing care of the total individual rather than concentrating on physical condition only. She was a member of the original staff of Hillhaven Hospice in Tucson, Arizona, and is now director of education at Hospice of the Valley in Phoenix, Arizona.

his psychoemotional and spiritual needs requires special skills and consumes more time.

Probably the most significant contribution emerging from the hospice concept is the relief of pain. As we know, pain wears many disguises and does not always have a physical basis.

Spiritual distress can greatly exacerbate physical pain. Conversely, unremitting physical pain can totally distract the terminally ill from responding to their spiritual needs. The reluctance and inability of many to deal with the spiritual inclinations of the terminally ill suggest the need to explore this dimension further.

Under the best conditions, a person cannot always articulate what he experiences in the depths of his being. Through introspection he may perceive subtle changes but be unable to explain the mysterious energy that at one time gently moves him in one direction and then another or swiftly carries him on a course that both frightens and fascinates him. It is not unusual for the terminally ill to share a spiritual experience in which they allude in some way to this inexplicable current.

The basic structure of the spiritual life is founded on a deep appreciation of the many levels of an individual's awareness. Unique to the hospice setting is the philosophy of providing an atmosphere in which the person may live fully and experience life on a variety of levels. To look beyond the physical needs of the terminally ill to an appreciation of the spiritual is to assure the individual that every effort will be made to provide the peace of mind that is fundamental to death with dignity.

The spiritual component of the personality is bound up in relationships—the relationship to self, to others, and to God. The latter two seem to require more resolution for the person who is faced with imminent death.

The work of the person whose life is measured in weeks or months is to resolve problems of relationships. To work with the terminally ill also involves the establishment of relationships between the sick person and the caregiver. The caregiver gently counsels and lovingly guides the sick person to a greater awareness of his relationships with himself, others, and God.

Sometimes family relationships that have suffered estrangement for years become critically important when a family member is faced with a terminal illness. One woman, estranged from her adult son and daughter for years, had been at hospice for four months when, following many hours of therapeutic conversation, she was able to effect a reconciliation with her children. The day following the reconciliation, when a nurse visiting the patient observed an open suitcase on the adjacent empty bed, the nurse attempted to close the suitcase and put it away when the patient said, "Not yet, nurse." The interdisciplinary hospice care team believed the request of the patient was symbolic that closure with her children was yet to take place. The following evening the son and daughter spent many hours with their mother in what appeared to be serious dialogue. Some forty-eight hours later the patient died with peace and dignity. Her son later said the three of them had been able to bring a peaceful closure to a long-broken relationship.

A person's relationship with God is not only an intriguing but also a mysterious one; it is the well-spring of his total spiritual life.

The relationship between patient and caregiver is one of giving and receiving. The caregiver must guard against assuming the role of beneficent giver. Unless the sick person is allowed to reciprocate in some way, the one-sided relationship will wane and die.

Caring for and sharing with the terminally ill has both physical and spiritual aspects. In caring for another, the giver helps the sick person become more aware of the mysterious dynamics at work in his life. The caregiver must provide time for the person to sort out his feelings, freedom to respond in the manner he chooses, and understanding and acceptance of where he is with regard to his impending death.

A demonstration of compassionate understanding and acceptance permits the terminally ill person to exercise his inner freedom to share himself, to close the door gently or to slam shut the secret chamber of his soul. An overzealous caregiver, in his desire to help, may find himself rushing in with a vehemence that militates against his ability to listen actively and to understand the dying person's painful message. Such behavior creates the potential of programming the life of the terminally ill and of imposing the caregiver's own will and needs into the world of the dying person.

To create a world of quiet and repose for the terminally ill is also to still the turbulent flood of one's own anxieties about dying and death.

Generally, interpersonal relationships are built on the foundation of human communication. A common ground is identified and a distinctive vocabulary is laid down. The degree of fulfillment one derives from the relationship is in direct proportion to the time and effort expended in learning to communicate on different levels. In the spiritual realm the relationship is between the individual and God. The usual manner of communication is called prayer.

Basic characteristics of meaningful communication in friendship are openness and trust. A person's prayer life should share the same characteristics. Frequently, the terminally ill person lacks the strength and energy to enter into deep prayer. In fact, the patient may even express an inability to focus his attention ever so briefly on a spiritual thought. Such a predicament can give rise to feelings of unworthiness and thoughts that God is no longer in his life. It is quite logical, then, for the clergy to become involved with the terminally ill person as early as possible. Trust, confidence, and fearless openness on the part of both the dying person and clergy which is established in timely fashion and sustained throughout the illness can be most helpful as the sick person grapples with problems perceived in his spiritual life.

If a close relationship between patient and clergy exists prior to the terminal illness, the patient will more readily look to his clergyman for the courage and strength he may receive through sympathetic and compassionate pastoral counseling.

Without betraying any confidence, the clergyman can be of invaluable assistance to the interdisciplinary team. Through better understanding of the strengths of patient and family, the team can develop more realistic plans for meeting all the family's needs.

The family may exhibit greater anxiety and concern than the dying person himself. The clergy should be invited to plan religious services in which the family participates, whether the loved one is in a hospice facility or in the hospice home-care program.

Although the clergy are especially equipped by their calling to utilize spiritual resources in certain crises, all members of a hospice team are encouraged to pray with the dying person and family if requested to do so.

An organized system of referrals maintains the spiritual link among the dying person, family, and clergy. The prayer of one's heart, although burdened with pain and sadness, can grow strong and courageous within the boundaries of a caring community. Together, family and hospice team can reach out beyond human limitations to offer each the freedom and space to be.

Sometimes a caregiver and a terminally ill person perceive the existence of a uniquely mysterious relationship. In comfortable silence they find themselves sharing a special part of themselves. Each encounter strengthens the spiritual bonds between them. Then one day the dying person trustingly parts the curtains of his spiritual domain and allows the other to perceive what is known only to God. This rare and treasured gift imposes special obligations on the recipient, and whether or not he realizes it at the time, his own spiritual life acquires a new dimension.

When the sick person enters into the dying process the experience is one of profound peace for both himself and his spiritual brother or sister. The relationship is intensified, and there is no longer a need to communicate with words. Touch is important in communication. Hands locked in a gentle living-dying clasp maintain a certain reality orientation. When eye contact is possible, volumes are spoken. An occasional verbal prayer or reassurance to the dying person that he is not alone dispels any thoughts of abandonment. When the final moment arrives for death to make its claim, the immediate environment is dignified by the peaceful fulfillment of the dying person in his "final stage of growth."

It is not uncommon for the terminally ill to express certain wishes in anticipation of the day of death. On one occasion a resident asked her

family to tape a Sunday service at her church and keep it available for
the day of her death. The family complied and on the day the resident
seemed ready to die the tape was played. The prayers and songs the resident had so often enjoyed through participation brought peace and fulfillment at death.

Staff members should be careful not to impose their own spiritual
values on hospice residents, but should rather permit them the "spiritual
space" they need for growth and/or resolution.

A person's relationship with God is considered too personal and sacred
to permit probing or trespassing.

Sometimes a family member will write a poem or prayer to be read
during the funeral service of a loved one, such as this poem a husband
wrote about his beloved wife:

> The star is passing on to
> the world of just beyond.
> The star you followed many nights
> and wondered where it was.
> The heavenly star is waiting for you,
> and will receive you with open arms.
> You've filled your earthly wants, and
> the star is waiting for you.
> Waiting patiently, and the star is
> grateful to receive you.

The poem was read by his minister during his wife's funeral service. This
personal contribution was a source of great comfort to him during
bereavement.

People relate to prayer during illness much as they did during health.
For some prayer is a vehicle for supplication, praise, and thanksgiving.
For others it is a delightful period of intimacy, a time when acceptance of
death is best reflected in this poem, *Twilight,* written about two weeks
prior to the woman's death:

**Twilight**

> The quietness of the hour
> And colored sky
> Bring thoughts which may be likened
> To the faint aroma of the wildest flower.
>
> Who has not seen the beauty thus exposed
> In this most hallowed hour
> Will never know
> The eternal magic of the day.

To know when to pray with the terminally ill and when to remain respectfully quiet comes with sensitivity not only to timing but to human need.

### SUPPORTING INDIVIDUAL LIFESTYLE THROUGH SOCIAL WORK SERVICES

Social work services are important to the multidisciplinary approach of supporting the personal integrity of people using hospice. Social services help the client and family to maintain meaningful personal relationships, and opportunities for continuity of social roles sustain access to needed resources and connect the individual with those individuals, groups, or systems that are needed to maintain dignified social living (Miller and Solomon, 1979).

The social worker may meet with the dying patient, with the patient and family, or with the family alone to assist with the mutual tasks as the patient approaches death. The patient and family need to cope with the illness, the anticipated death, and the changing social organization of the family.

The dying person needs to be surrounded by caring people and to continue to deal with the realities of life and the end of life. Disguised responses on the part of family may create additional discomfort. The family group can be helped to deal with improving communications among family members; helped to reminisce about good times; and helped to support continuing family activities that enhance the role of the dying person through celebrations, parties, visits with friends, and maintenance of enjoyable activities.

Multifamily groups become an important tool to build new supports for families, which through them can share experiences with others facing a similar crisis. New caring relationships may ease stress through exchanged expressions of concern and awareness of comparable problems.

The social worker, intervening and helping in the resolution of problems, increasing communications, and maintaining the family organization, helps maintain the dignity of the individual and his ability to cope. The dying person still wants to be regarded by others as worthy. He needs to know that he will be missed and that the family will survive.

Those who reside in the inpatient hospice environment have opportunities to observe and react to the way dying and death are treated in the institutional environment. Each individual learns of his own potential fate, and each death becomes an anticipation or rehearsal of his own dying. Individuals prepare for anticipated trauma by rehearsing, in the mind, the sequence of events and consequences and the responses of others related to them. By reviewing and sorting out the situation, the "worry work" becomes productive because it provides a rehearsal for coming events. The social worker can assist in this rehearsal by observing with the patient the events occurring in hospice and the reactions of staff and family. The patient should observe that life and death both are respected, that death is dealt with openly, and that the wishes of each individual are carefully observed. The social worker can help the patient determine how he wants his own death to be handled and how he can maintain mastery over his own life in the process.

### SUPPORTING INDIVIDUAL LIFESTYLE THROUGH CREATIVE COMMUNICATIONS

"Creative communications" is the term chosen to describe a prototype program developed by Barry Rogers (1978) at Hillhaven Hospice in Tucson. Here, the arts are used to enable patients to express their needs, anxieties, and fears, as well as to communicate a sense of perspective in reviewing their lives. Painting, music, and poetry are some of the arts introduced into the program and experiencing them seems to be important to patients for whom traditional counseling seems inappropriate.

Similar programs, under the direction of persons who combine talent in the arts with a capacity for bringing out the creativity of others, can greatly enhance the lives of hospice residents and help them express feelings that are important to them.

### SUPPORTING INDIVIDUAL LIFESTYLES THROUGH HUMOR

Even in response to the needs of the dying person there is a place for humor; it helps make dying a part of the total living experience. Reminiscing about humorous events in life as part of a reflection of life can add comfort and open communications with the dying person. The ability of the dying person to deal with humor, if it is in keeping with the lifestyle of the person, is also an opportunity for maintaining control, as is illustrated in the following anecdote:

> An old woman was dying at home, and at the moment when she was apparently about to die she was in bed, head propped upon some pillows, eyes closed. A large number of her family were standing around in stony silence waiting for her death. The old woman opened her eyes, scanned the scene, and softly said, "A watched pot never boils."

Some new humor has come out of the hospice movement. For example, where staff find family, patient, or visitors creating problems and becoming anxious and resistant to requests, the staff comment may be a suggestion "to offer them a Brompton's cocktail and they'll do anything you request."

Hospice is different from other institutions because pets often are accepted there. Knowing this, a hospice patient asked the administrator if he could bring his pet into the building. The administrator responded that it was in keeping with the hospice policies and that if it was important to the patient it was acceptable to hospice. The patient repeated the question to be assured of the response and he was again told it was permissible to bring the pet into the hospice building. Several moments later the administrator was surprised to find several friends escorting the patient's pet donkey through the corridors of the building.

Humorous stories are also used to poke fun at some of the traditional professional roles in health care as is illustrated in the following story told by a hospice employee.

A young man died after a brief illness and was rewarded by going to heaven. When he arrived and was greeted by a host of nurse-angels, he was startled and disoriented. He made some inquiries about the setting and then asked whether he had died.

The nurse-angels were obviously flustered and asked the young man if he had discussed this with his physician.

## Hospice Concept Is More Than Bricks and Mortar

In its total organization, hospice not only serves its users but makes a strong statement to the community that there can be a better way to provide care to dying persons. To those who will never use or need hospice, it symbolizes an important concept in overcoming the fear accompanying death from cancer. While hospice does not promise the prolongation of life nor the cure of cancer, it does promise a concept of caring and dealing with death while preventing pain.

Hospice also makes a statement about the conscious acceptance of death as part of life. While the subtitle of hospice need not, crudely, label it a death house, it must be acknowledged that people who enter into a hospice program do so with the awareness that death is imminent. But in hospice death can be dealt with as part of life.

**Principle:**  *Hospice care requires home-care services and the capability of providing institutional care.*

**Discussion:**  Can a hospice program be designed and contemplated without a building? Because the ability to provide suitable home care is often dependent upon the backup resource of an inhouse program, a resident facility is probably essential. Home care is made more viable when institutional care can be readily available, offering the same concepts and philosophy of caring and assuring that the client will be admitted immediately, not placed on a waiting list for the next available bed somewhere.

Can hospice care be provided in a residential center alone? That, too, would compromise the basic philosophy. If the dying person wishes to remain at home for as long as possible and only the residential hospice is available, he is robbed of one of the essential choices. He cannot control his life if his choice becomes so limited.

Can hospice care be provided in a hospital? It can if hospice care is indeed differentiated from acute care and if the other levels of care are available to provide the full hospice continuum.

Can hospice care be provided in a long-term care setting? Again, the answer is yes if the care provided is hospice care rather than chronic care and if the full continuum is available.

In summary, hospice care can be provided in a variety of different settings and environments. It is not the building or the program title that defines the program. The essential elements are the content of the program and the continuum of multiple levels of care. Of equal importance is the special role of staff, who share the goals and recognize the character of hospice care. Where hospice is provided as a unit within another institutional setting, i.e., a hospital or nursing home, it is essential that hospice maintain its own administrative structure, staffing, schedules, and priorities in order to maintain the uniqueness of its program and competence of its staff to provide hospice care.

## Continuum of Care

Hospice supports the contention that many people would choose to die at home if the appropriate supports were available. With the caution offered that we not assume the individual's preference but rather learn the preference from direct inquiry, it may not always be possible to keep the individual at home. In some situations the individual may be permitted to remain at home because of the availability of the inpatient facility, the supports it offers, the respite care available, and the option of not using the hospital emergency room at times of heightened stress or crisis. All of the hospice services need to be integrated into a comprehensive program so that when the person is accepted for care, there is acceptance into a total program.

**Principle:** *The full continuum of hospice care should include home care, day and night care, inpatient care, and bereavement services. These* *services should be coordinated in a comprehensive continuum having a single administrative structure and a coordinated intake process.*

**Discussion:** Inherent in the hospice concept is the recognition that rapid changes take place in the individual's and family's capacities to cope, which are affected by remission as well as by crises. When multiple levels of care are available, the intensity of service as well as the location of the provision of service can be varied and modified to meet individual needs. Hospice has characteristics of an emergency system built into its design, but these are not the acute care, lifesaving responses of the hospital emergency room.

*Inpatient care* within the institutional facility on a twenty-four-hour-a-day basis is the proper alternative once it has been ascertained that an acute care facility is inappropriate. The physican may refer to inpatient hospice for care because cure is no longer the appropriate goal, if the patient has distressing symptoms that cannot be managed at home, or if he needs skilled care which cannot be provided there. When the patient is cared for at home, a close relationship must exist with an inpatient facility which can offer twenty-four-hour nursing care in the event that the person giving care at home becomes ill or for some other reason cannot continue to function. Supportive services can be made available at the hospice

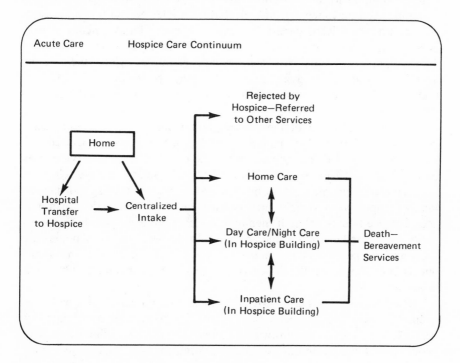

**Figure 4–2** Continuum of Hospice Care

on very short notice whenever the family cannot handle the situation at home. When family relationships are strained or difficult, the added burden of illness may create overwhelming problems. Admitting the person to the inpatient facility can sometimes salvage a threatened relationship, providing the patient and his family a respite from the burden of guilt and other defenses brought on by the complex situation.

*Home health services* are the part of a hospice program which provides care for patients and support for their families in their own homes. Nursing, occupational and physical therapies, dietary counseling, social work, medical and pharmaceutical services, and spiritual services are provided in the home as they are needed. Home health services take professional health services into the dwelling place of the dying person, helping him to remain independent. Patients can remain at home in familiar surroundings, with their independence limited only by their frailty. Remaining at home increases the patient's sense of control over his own life and permits him to make decisions and choices. Many ethnic groups believe that care of a relative must be provided in the home rather than in an institution unless acute care is required. Such wishes and beliefs must be respected.

In other family situations, it may be easier for the family to have the patient admitted to an institution than to organize care at home. Such a decision may lead to feelings of guilt that must later be confronted. Awareness of how the dying person is treated by other family members may affect children who, of course, observe how their parents treat terminally ill grandparents. Home care can provide resources which help family members sustain their dying relative. It must be recognized, however, that maintenance of a person at home may not always be in the best interest of everyone involved.

Ongoing evaluation of the patient, family members, and other caregivers is necessary so that changes that take place may be recognized and evaluated. Care of dying persons is not static and additional services may be required as the patient's condition, or family ability to cope, changes.

Home care has the dual purpose of providing care plus supporting the family's capacity to remain the primary caregiver. To accomplish this goal, hospice home-care staff members use each visit as a teaching opportunity to strengthen family members' skills. In some hospice home-care programs the home visit is conducted by two staff persons so that while one is providing care the other is assisting family members with their responsibilities.

Home-care services are provided on an intermittent basis, with frequency of each type of help assessed by the home-care coordinator as part of the ongoing monitoring of care. During the initial assessment period and when symptom control is a problem, staff may make daily visits with more frequent phone calls. Frequency of visits may also be increased when the patient or family requires more intensive emotional support.

Daily visits may also be required for teaching the patient or caregiver a new procedure.

When the person dies at home, some member of the home-care team will go to the home and remain with the family until the body is removed. One staff member will be assigned as the bereavement counselor, will attend the funeral services, and do follow-up assessments and counseling as needed at the end of a week, one month, three months, six months, and a year.

The home-care program regularly operates from Monday through Friday from 8:30 A.M. to 5 P.M. On call availability is provided after hours and on weekends and holidays by registered nurses from the program.

Volunteers may perform a variety of tasks, including doing errands, providing transportation, helping with light household chores, friendly visiting, giving bereavement support and counseling, helping to mobilize resources from the community, and offering clerical assistance in the home-care office. Home-care meetings should be held weekly and be led by the home-care coordinator. All staff members and volunteers should attend.

The usual agenda might consist of:

· Announcements, information sharing.
· Patient and family review, including bereavement activities.
· Discussion of deaths with an evaluation of care provided to patients and family.
· Completion of problem-oriented progress notes.
· Review and revision of care plans.
· Discussion of goals, policies, practices, scope of services, and community relationships.*

*Day care or night care* can provide all the hospice services to a patient when key family members can no longer be in attendance twenty-four hours a day. In day care, the patient may be brought to the hospice facility for several hours each day during which he receives food, medication, lodging, and nursing care. Family members or other caretakers, meanwhile, can be temporarily relieved of their care responsibilities and have time for socialization, business, or just time off. The patient returns to his home for the night. Alternatively, night care can be provided within the hospice if that is the kind of relief from constant attention to the ill person that will be most helpful.

By providing a combination of resident and nonresident services, the

* Adapted from Hillhaven Hospice home-care program.

hospice program is able to vary appropriately both the quantity and quality of services supplied. Patients can remain with their families for part of the day, evening, or night, with hospice services complementing the home care and giving respite to family or other caregivers. Day or night care services also may make it possible for patients who live alone and can manage during the day or during the night but not for a twenty-four-hour period to maintain greater independence. Transportation may be provided by the family, by the hospice program, or by a community transportation system. The flexibility of this program aids both patients and those involved with them. By having it, hospice clearly demonstrates that the services offered are designed to meet the varied needs of the recipients of care, the patients and their families.

*Bereavement services* are provided to families and/or those responsible for care after the death of a patient. Part of care of the dying is care of the survivors. It can also be comforting to the dying person to know that the family will not be left uncared for. Bereavement follow-up is actually preventive health care. In the first year after the loss of a family member or other intimate, there is increased vulnerability to illness for the survivor, who also may be susceptible to increased drug ingestion (including that of alcohol) and/or depression. Visits to the bereaved, offering counseling and support, should be made available for a period of one year after the patient's death or until it is clear that the services are no longer needed.

The dying person and his family are the core of concern for the hospice team. When the patient dies, the death itself changes the locus of attention from the deceased to the survivors. There may be both an outpouring of emotions and an unquestionable sigh of relief that the suffering is over and the traumatic part of life is ended. Survivors are not at first exposed to the loss and loneliness because of the focus on myriad details involving financial matters as well as relating to family members and visitors. Families and friends converge—where survivors are fortunate to have these concerned persons—but all at the same time. Then the visitors leave and the supports are reduced. It is at this time that hospice services reach out to the bereaved to complete the program of care.

Grief is the expression most often used to characterize the survivor's distressed state. Mourning, on the other hand, refers to the culturally patterned manner of expressing the response to death. Styles of mourning vary with culture, religion, and background; they also change with time. Specific styles of mourning are associated with ethnic groups, but even these change over the years. In one study, Fulton (1976) reports that those persons who minimized the ceremonies of mourning a year later had increased depression and anxiety and used more drugs and alcohol. When cremation had taken place, serious disturbances among the bereaved appear to have been more common than among those who experienced the process of burial and mourning.

In our contemporary society, the mourners are urged to return to a state of normalcy as quickly as possible, cutting short the period of grief and mourning. It is important to note that mourning, in most cases, lasts for at least a year and that rushing its completion may prolong or intensify the entire process. It is for this reason that bereavement services should be available for that length of time. There is evidence to suggest that the traditional Irish wake or the Jewish shiva (culturally prescribed rituals following death) contribute to good mental health. Grief is a necessary reaction to loss and is not a sign of weakness or self-indulgence. Funerals and other rituals make death a reality as well as bring support and warmth to the bereaved person through the attention and concern of family and friends (Fiefel, 1977).

In several Hispanic cultures there is the ritual of *velorio,* which is similar to the Irish wake. This is the time when family and friends gather after the patient's death to view the body. They serve food and drink, reminisce, cry, and pray. Another custom often observed in Hispanic cultures is a nine-day period of prayers in church or at home known as *novenario.* During this period members of the extended family make bereavement visits among their members. The Roman Catholic faith and Hispanic culture serve to permit the outpouring of feeling and encourage the assembling of loved ones so that emotions can be publicly and freely expressed. This permits the social support system of the extended family to operate (Kalish and Reynolds, 1976).

The grief an individual may feel before the death of a loved one is known as anticipatory grief and may mitigate the post-mortem grief. Persons experience grief symptoms in response to the expected loss and then may have an abbreviated reaction upon actual loss. However, the dying person must die before the bereaved can actually respond to death and redefine a new lifestyle. It appears that some degree of anticipatory grief occurs for all expected losses and hospice staff should understand that physical or emotional withdrawal or apparently callous responses may be evidence of anticipatory grief. It is important for hospice staff to know that grief begins from the moment a family member is told that the patient is not likely to recover.

Listening to the concerns and observing the reaction of the family is part of meeting the patient's needs. Offering support without being judgmental is often the key to providing care. A family may look for a scapegoat upon whom to blame their misfortune. They may be angry. Careful listening without arguing, rationalizing, or becoming defensive is usually the most helpful approach. Encouraging family members to assist with the patient's care and praising their efforts is still another way of helping them grieve (Lamerton, 1973).

The typical features of grief are described in three stages: 1) shock, characterized by numbness and lasting from a few hours to several weeks;

2) marked mental anguish, during which aimlessness and depression may be experienced for a period lasting from three to ten weeks; and 3) developing awareness, in which sadness, hopelessness, helplessness, and emptiness are followed by a recovery in which accommodations are made and new relationships are established. Recovery is most difficult for older survivors, for whom new associations, opportunities for socialization, and new interpersonal relations may be limited.

During the period of intense grief soon after the death, the overwhelming need is usually for empathy and strong emotional support. In the later stages of bereavement, the survivor's needs shift toward assistance in returning to a normal social life. In his book *Bereavement,* Dr. Colin Murray Parks (1972) points out that the role of the hospice staff member doing bereavement work is difficult and inevitably involves pain. This cannot be avoided because it stems from the awareness of both parties that neither can give the other what he wants. The helper (counselor) cannot bring back the person who is dead, and the bereaved person cannot gratify the helper by seeming helped.

The bereaved may review the time before the death for evidence of others' failure to be helpful to the dead family member. Some may accuse themselves of negligence or exaggerate minor omissions. These problems can be mitigated by visits from a hospice staff member who listens to the survivor without criticism of any expressions of guilt. The bereaved can thus discover it is safe to let out pent-up feelings and is then free to get on with the grief work.

Working with bereaved families may also require helping family members to continue traditional signs of mourning for the sake of the survivors and to maintain long-established cultural practices, i.e., wearing of special clothes or abstinence from some social activities.

A difficult time for a survivor is usually the first anniversary of the death. It is a time when support is needed and a visit from a hospice staff member is appropriate. Many cultures mark the one-year anniversary of the death of a loved one. It is often the time when "official" mourning ceases. For example, at the end of the year traditional Latin cultures permit the return to nonmourning clothes and the bereaved may attend social gatherings or remarry (Kalish and Reynolds, 1976).

It may be appropriate for the hospice staff to identify "high-risk" family members and to follow these persons more closely during the bereavement period. Another way of assisting survivors is to encourage their participation as volunteers in the hospice program. Many find that their burdens lift as they help others who are experiencing what they have gone through. This is usually helpful in overcoming depression in the final stage of grieving and often encourages the survivor to begin to take on a new role.

While all hospice staff persons are involved in bereavement work if they have any contact with patient or family, it is important to clarify staff responsibility for bereavement services. This component of care may be coordinated by the social worker or chaplain and may call for a standing staff committee that regularly reviews the bereavement program and assures that every bereaved family has a support service available.

The skilled volunteer, especially one who may have experienced the death of someone in hospice, may provide an important resource for bereavement follow-up, referring more troubled families to the social work staff.

Many of the bereavement services can be carried out through groups, classes, and social programs. For example, a regularly scheduled meeting for relatives of hospice patients provides an opportunity for peer group associations, supports, and personal contacts. There is need for assistance with some of the confusing details of insurance, Medicare, Social Security, wills and estates, taxes, etc., and these can be handled in small classes specifically designed to deal with these problems of survivorship. Representatives of the insurance industry, lawyers and legal aid societies, and accountants are good persons to provide some of the necessary information. Social gatherings, picnics, and parties, especially around holidays, provide an informal setting for people to share problems, identify continuing need for services, and strengthen the social support network. Parties can be fun and may help those needing help to reach out for it.

Bereaved families may also need opportunities to thank hospice staff members for their kindness and caring. It may be too difficult to expect that families will feel welcomed at hospice unless a special effort is made. A family meeting or a phone call to the bereaved may be the best way to invite a visit. For the bereaved, the ability to communicate appreciation may be an important aspect of the bereavement, as it defines a sense of closure to the care experience.

## Organization of Hospice Care

A continuum can be defined as a sequence of things in a regular order. A continuum of care in a hospice program includes many levels of care, ranging from the most intensive, which usually takes place in the inpatient setting, to supportive services when the patient and family need minimal assistance. Along the continuum are the services discussed at greater length in the previous sections: inpatient care, day care, night care, home care, and bereavement services.

**Principle:** *The most efficient and humanely responsive way to offer services is to provide a single point of entry into the program. This should begin with an assessment and intake procedure during which a coordinator* *or facilitator assesses the family, the patient, and their combined resources and limitations. The facilitator's role should always be that of an advocate for the patient. The assessment should take place immediately after the referral from a physician is made and should include an assurance to the patient and family that if hospice is selected as the appropriate setting for that patient's care, it stands ready to provide services twenty-four hours a day.*

**Discussion:** *Assessment and Intake.* The continuum must begin with a procedure by which it can be determined whether or not hospice is the best care program available for the person involved. Hospice may not be the best program for all dying persons.

The following are situations where hospice care may not be appropriate:

1. The dying person and/or family are not able to deal with the dying process and find hospice too threatening to be helpful.
2. The applicant may be too close to death to justify a move into another care setting or change in the routine of care he is receiving.
3. The individual and family are content with the care currently being received.
4. The cost of hospice care or limits of insurance coverage or benefits from other third-party payers put hospice care beyond the financial means of the patient and family.

Inquiries and referrals to hospice care may be received from physicians, nurses, discharge planners, ministers, friends, relatives, or the patient himself, who may have learned of the program through relatives, personal experiences, community promotion, or publicity. However, in all cases, the acceptance of a person into hospice care is dependent upon the approval and support of a physician. Hospice care cannot be offered without the involvement and leadership of the physician as a critical member of the hospice team.

**Table 4–1** Criteria for Acceptance into Hospice

1. Patient has a diagnosis of a terminal illness.
2. The disease is determined to be beyond the state of aggressive treatment for cure; however, palliative treatment for symptom control is acceptable.
3. The patient and family wish to enter the hospice program.
4. General life expectancy is less than six months.
5. The personal physician agrees to the referral and will continue to attend the patient.
6. A competent caregiver is available to the patient in the home if home care is recommended.

Application for hospice care should be considered for the total program, not for one of its components. The applicant accepted for hospice care should be assigned to the appropriate level of care at the time of admission, based on the needs of the applicant and the resources of hospice.

The primary site for providing hospice care is the individual's own home. Maintaining the patient in the household is dependent upon the functional status of the individual and the support structure of the family, the household, and neighbors. The assessment for hospice care must, therefore, include evaluation of the individual's social support structure, which oftentimes extends beyond or outside of the family. A thorough appraisal of the physical characteristics of the household, with recommendations for adjustments enhancing the possibility of caring for the individual at home, is essential before any recommendations for home care can be made.

Evaluating an applicant for the continuum of hospice care, and promoting the concept of hospice as a continuum, implies the availability of every level of care for each participant. Should a dying person and his family apply for hospice care, with physician support, and specifically request the inpatient level of care, careful assessment might make it clear that the applicant is a good candidate for hospice care who could be supported comfortably at home, although the family exhibits a high level of anxiety. Such a family should be encouraged to care for the person at home for as long as possible, postponing the use of the institution's re-

**Table 4–2**  Admission Process for Hospice Care

1. Referral is directed to the intake facilitator from patient, family, physician, or hospital.
2. Facilitator gathers clinical data (from attending physician, hospital records, etc.), family and personal data, financial information (from patient/family), and completes a preadmission worksheet.
3. Facilitator makes initial judgment that patient is eligible for hospice program. If patient is not admitted to hospice, referral is made to an appropriate agency.
4. Appropriate level of hospice care (home care, inpatient care, etc.) is determined from clinical data and patient desires and is reviewed by a multidisciplinary team (intake facilitator, care coordinator, physician, social worker).
5. After decision is made to admit to hospice and the care level has been determined, the collected information is forwarded to either the inpatient or home-care coordinator, who then initiates the care plan.
6. Coordinator consults patient's attending physician for orders and approval of initial care plan.
7. Care plan is instituted and regularly reviewed by the multidisciplinary care team (medical director, nursing staff, facilitator, care coordinator, social worker).

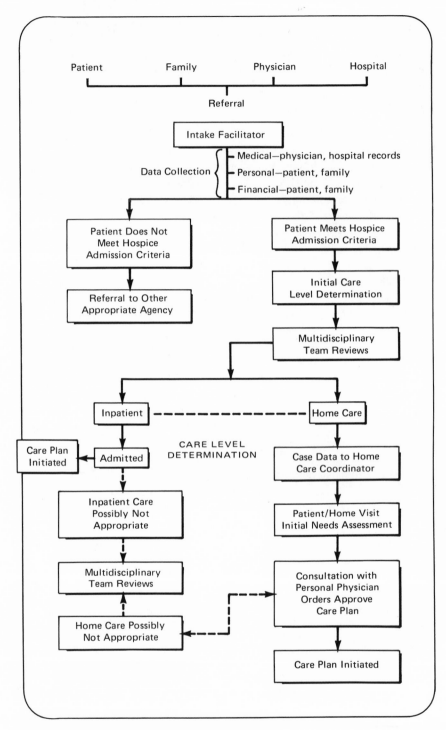

**Figure 4–3** Hospice Admission Procedures

*Source:* Adapted from Dr. Steven Cox, Medical Director, Hillhaven Hospice Home Care Program, Tucson, Arizona.

sources until home support is no longer adequate. A promise and commitment that the institutional care will be available when needed must, of course, be made and honored. It is important that new families be admitted into the hospice system only when there is assurance that the entire system can be responsive to the patient's needs.

*Gatekeeper or Facilitator Function.* An important part of the continuum is the gatekeeping function that coordinates the service functions with the needs of participants. Whether the function is labeled "gatekeeper," "case manager," "facilitator," or any other name is not important, but this function must be performed. Essentially, what is required is that one staff person, having an overview of the total system, coordinate the services for each participant, assuring that within the system he is neither underserved nor overserved. The case manager, while not directly involved in providing care, maintains an overview of the progression of services without having to defend or justify his own service function. The case manager can assess the household, evaluate the social support network, and provide the coordinating function—especially important in sustaining a person at home.

The case manager is the facilitator for the individual using the continuum of hospice care. The case manager assures the continuity of care and the capacity of the continuum to meet the changing needs.

*Twenty-Four-Hour Coverage.* While it is perfectly clear that twenty-four-hour service is provided in the institutional environment, the same continuity of coverage must be provided to support care of the dying person at home. Anxiety in those persons providing home care often is related to the uncertainty of receiving needed supports at night, on weekends, and on holidays. Hospice has to assure the availability of the twenty-four-hour support system and should carefully instruct the participant on how to use the system. If emergency phone calls are to be routed through the institutional setting, relationships among hospice staff should be described. Where an electronic call system is used, prompt response in relaying a phone message must be assured.

Early experiences in hospice home-care programs have demonstrated that there have been few evening calls, and these often can be appropriately dealt with on the phone. This is so, however, where the hospice staff has been thorough in teaching the family and patient, where there has been a clear understanding of expectations and resources, and where hospice staff has communicated its caring and availability.

*Single Point of Entry.* Although the hospice system may become far-reaching in the number of people served and the variety of locations of home care, inpatient care, and other services, it is essential to maintain a single point of entry into the system. This central point of control is essential to assure that the total hospice program will be available to each applicant from the moment he is accepted for care.

Finally, it should be noted that applicants for hospice service and participants in the program are prone to be depleted of physical energies and need to focus on the end of life opportunities rather than the bureaucracy of any caring system. The hospice continuum of care, the evaluation, the case manager's role, and all the other characteristics of the continuum are built into the system to ease the trauma for the dying person and family. The organizational structure is required to assure the proper delivery of hospice care and to minimize the problems and red tape of transfers from one level of care to another. Once a patient has been admitted into the hospice system, all energies must be directed to the appropriate care for the dying person and his family. The organizational structure must never become self-serving or imitate those of other modes of care for traditional values alone. Hospice care is based on the urgency of need, the limited time available, and the potential crisis for individual and family. The management plan must assure that these needs are kept in focus at all times and that the dying person is understood to be the only reason the organization exists. The organizational behavior must continue to represent this ideal.

## Privacy

The concept of privacy is closely related to individual dignity and the continuing role of the family. The issue of privacy is of special importance in the institutional environment, where privacy may be difficult to assure. Interestingly, there is no conflict between the need for privacy and the need not to be left alone. The essential ingredient is respect for choice and control.

**Principle:** *Privacy in the inpatient facility should be provided in response to the needs and desires of individuals and their families.*

**Discussion:** When the dying person wants to be alone or be with people of his own choice, that option should be available in the hospice inpatient environment. That option can be provided by having private rooms or shared rooms in conjunction with family rooms where the person can retreat from the "sick" room environment to a living room, sitting room, or bedroom furnished in a "homelike" manner, having both warmth and comfort.

The desire not to be alone may not be met by sharing a room with one or more other dying persons. The person seeking companionship is looking for support and comfort directed specifically to his needs and well-being. Other hospice clients may not have the personal strength or forebearance to succor a roommate or neighbor. They may be seeking a giving relationship that is focused on their own needs.

Providing privacy also may test staff sensitivity to individual needs and differences. Knocking on the door before entering a room gives evidence of a respect for privacy. Encouraging the patient to surround himself with special mementos and manipulating the environment for the individual's comfort may be appropriate behavior to establish a sense of privacy. Staff recognition of personal needs, protection of individual possessions, and respect for personal space preserve the dignity of the individual and give support to the positive aspects of the hospice environment.

The special attractiveness of hospice care as a demonstration of the humanizing of care of the dying within the health care system has made it the focus of considerable community attention. Many groups and individuals want to observe or study hospice care. While this community interest should be encouraged, it cannot be permitted to interfere with the privacy needs of hospice patients. Inpatient hospice programs should establish a committee to sort out requests for visits or tours and establish policies that afford the privacy required, while still maintaining positive community relations. It is important for patients and families to serve on this committee along with staff.

## Personal Belongings

Hospice differs from the other environments that focus on caring for the sick by striving to enable the individual to live as fully as possible for whatever remaining time he has left. The positive qualities of living should be stressed, and within the institutional environment, every effort should be made to create a warm, homelike atmosphere. The furniture, furnishings, selection of colors, and decor should communicate that hospice is a setting for living. Display of personal belongings should be invited by window ledges, shelves, and tackable wall surfaces. There should be open floor space for a favorite chair.

**Principle:**   *The patient should be encouraged to bring personal items and belongings to the inpatient facility and should be provided space to use and display them.*

**Discussion:**   Many health care facilities discourage bringing personal belongings cherished by the patient into the institution because of the burden it places on the institution if items are lost or stolen. Elaborate procedures are developed to insure the security of personal belongings.

There is no question that encouraging people to bring their personal items with them entails risk, but the comfort, and even joy, derived from doing so is worth it.

It seems especially important that religious items such as pictures or statues, as well as family pictures and greeting cards, have a place to be displayed within view and reach.

The important personal attachment to pets should not have to be severed by entering into the hospice facility. Provision should be made for pets to be brought regularly for visits if it is not possible for the pet to move into the hospice facility, taking into account the rights of other occupants and the type of pet and its behavior.

## Food and Dining

Typically in our society, foods are associated with the special events in life. Birthdays and birthday cakes are synonymous. Receptions become part of the festivity involved in a wedding, graduation, new job, or other special event. Taking a date out to dinner is an act of adulthood, and adults celebrate with friends or family with food.

Additionally, food is the sustenance of life, the source of energy and health. People eat to grow big and tall, to gain energy in order to work hard, to regain strength after illness.

For all these reasons, food is also important to people in hospice. It is associated with good health, and enjoyment of it is associated with building strength and energy to deal with the destructiveness of illness. Food also represents an association with good times, special events and reflecting on the good things in life, while at the same time it helps generate strength to deal with current traumas.

**Principle:**   *Food prepared in hospice should take into account the individual preferences of patients as well as their cultural practices.*

**Discussion:**   Food prepared in hospice should be unlike that typical of institutions. Cultural and ethnic foods and a variety of dishes will help people feel at home. Patients will let hospice staff know whether food is dull or interesting, and staff should listen. Food service should be scheduled so that participants can eat when they are in the mood and ready to eat. Loss of appetite is a frequent symptom of hospice clients and especially enticing foods should be available. The food service organization and method of delivery to participants should be flexible and tailored to meet unusual requirements. Because eating may be slow, hot food should be so served that it retains the heat for long periods; meals might be served in courses, with some dishes kept heated while others are being eaten. Food service is a strong and frequent signal about the special character of the hospice environment.

It is also important to provide the setting and support necessary to enable families to eat together in a private dining area. Having a food preparation area or a place to reheat and serve home-cooked food will encourage families to bring favorite foods to the hospice resident. In addition to the value this would have to the hospice resident, it becomes an important vehicle for the family to continue involvement in the care of their loved one. At times the family needs tangible ways to demonstrate concern. Preparation of a favorite meal and sharing that meal are such opportunities.

Hospice policies should also support staff's response to the unusual food request—unusual either in terms of the food request itself or in the time of the request. While all hospices may not be located adjacent to a food store open twenty-four hours each day, it is possible to freeze and store predictable favorites. Information about food likes or fetishes can be elicited during the orientation interview with the client and family.

With so many aspects in the care of the dying beyond the control of the caregiver, it behooves the hospice administration to assure that the food service will be most responsive to the individual needs of each patient. Staff should be directed to respond to these special requests as promptly as could reasonably be expected.

One woman recently admitted to a hospice inpatient facility was asked by the administrator if hospice could respond to any special request. The woman replied that her favorite dish was flamingo's tongue and she had not had any for a long time. Not to be daunted by this unusual request, the administrator searched the community and found a Chinese cook whose specialty was flamingo's tongue. The cook prepared a meal with all the trimmings for the woman and thanked hospice for the opportunity to meet this special request of a dying person.

## Limits on Restrictive Activities

Institutional health care environments are obliged to impose restrictions on their patients and visitors. The hours of visiting are controlled as is the number of visitors. Food intake, smoking, and the consumption of alcohol are carefully monitored. Pets are generally not welcome. Rules and regulations are written to enable staff to function in the most efficient manner to respond to the curative aspects of patient care. In contrast to the above, the organizational structure of hospice should be primarily focused on the needs, desires, and conveniences of the hospice user.

**Principle:**    *Hospice regulations should be held to a minimum and be related to life, safety, and licensing regulations. Hospice clients should enjoy the greatest flexibility and responsiveness to their own needs.*

**Discussion:**    Regulations or rules are necessary to protect the rights of all. Safety is also an important consideration. A patient who is drowsy may wish to smoke in bed. This can be permitted, but only if someone remains with him. Other rules may be made flexible in the same kind of way. In a like manner, the number or frequency of visits should not be regulated unless at the request of the patient. Visitors to patients should be welcome at all hours, and schedules should be oriented to the patient rather than to a predetermined work schedule.

It is important that all hospice rules be carefully reviewed to assess their impact on the caring environment, to determine their compatibility with the hospice philosophy, and to ascertain whether or not they are necessary in the hospice milieu. Patients who use the hospice facility should be encouraged to use it with the greatest possible flexibility and comfort.

## Summary

The hospice program has been described as the collective efforts of a multi-disciplinary caring team on behalf of the patient and his family. It can be offered at home as well as in an inpatient facility but it should be tailored to meet the individual patient's needs.

What people need when they are dying is relief from distressing symptoms, the presence of caring people, a comfortable environment, and the opportunity to continue to live in their own unique lifestyle until death. This requires respect for the individual's cultural and religious background as well as his role in family and community. It requires an understanding of the individual's self-perception and provision of the nutritive environment to sustain that person.

Whether services are delivered at home or in institutional settings, they should represent the hospice characteristics which include:

1. Coordinated care, including home care and inpatient services under a central administration offered in a continuum having centralized intake and case management.
2. Control of symptoms, including the physical, social, psychological, and spiritual manifestations of those symptoms.
3. Provision of care by a multidisciplinary team directed by a physician and including volunteers.
4. Availability of services on a twenty-four-hour-a-day, seven-day-a-week basis.

5. Consideration of the patient and family as the unit of care.
6. Provision of bereavement services.

In the context of a man's life, caring has a way of ordering his other values and activities around it. When this ordering is comprehensive, because of the inclusiveness of his caring, there is a basic stability in his life; he is "in place" in the world, instead of being out of place, or merely drifting or endlessly seeking his place. Through caring for certain others, by serving them through caring, a man lives in the meaning of his own life. In the sense in which a man can ever be said to be at home in the world, he is at home not through dominating, or explaining, or appreciating, but through caring and being cared for.

*Milton Mayeroff*

# 5

## *Staff*

Despite all of our modern medical terminology it is an
incontrovertible fact that each person who is born will
eventually die. The education of the health professional
does not prepare him to cope adequately either with
the needs of the dying patient, the needs of
the patient's family, or even his own reactions to
the death of his patient.

Jessie L. Steinfeld, M.D.

. . . *professional anxieties aroused in dealing with
catastrophic diseases and terminal illness are observable
phenomena for which a coping mechanism can
be developed. The social worker, or other professional,
who is helped to come to grips with his own
feelings is better able to give strength and support
to patients and relatives. The patient can be
helped to die with dignity and self-respect; families can
be helped to come through a traumatic experience with
some semblance of mental health.*

Bernice Catherine Harper

THE TWO QUOTES by Steinfeld and Harper readily expose the dilemma and reality for staff. Most staff are not prepared to deal with the work environment of death, yet staff can be helped to prepare for this important service. If hospice care is to be provided, it will be the service of a competent, trained staff. But what these quotes do not communicate is the special opportunities there are for people who work in hospice. It's not that being a member of a staff requires a special kind of person. Hospice personnel are like the people you find in most segments of health care. What is special are the responsibilities they have assumed to deliver this very personal quality of health care, combined with a responsibility to demonstrate hospice values to the community. What hospice staff has done is to step forward from the ranks and venture into something new. We know that change is generally associated with increased anxiety and uncertainty; hospice staffs have been able to assert themselves in spite of the uncertainties.

So what should be said is that in spite of modern medical technology that has separated personal care from the patient and despite the greater anxiety both in working with the terminally ill and in new situations, there has arisen a dedicated group of hospice personnel who are doing the caring we expect from them and hospice.

**Principle:** *Hospice staff must be carefully selected, trained, and supported to cope with the problems of working with dying patients and their families.*

**Discussion:** Contradicting a prediction that working in a hospice program would be depressing to staff and thus make it difficult to attract good people, hospice staff have been self-selected, positively attracted to providing care for the dying. Staff members proclaim that working in hospice is a fulfillment of their life goals, providing an opportunity for the expression of the deep concerns they have for others, a special trust and, therefore, a most rewarding experience. In some ways, hospice staff exhibit a missionary zeal, a religious expression of caring, and an intense feeling of involvement and commitment.

To what extent is this a reaction to the newness of hospice in our health care system? Does it reflect a disillusionment of staff with the large size of other sectors of health care? Will it wear off with the novelty of the experience?

The missionary zeal is undoubtedly a product of the newness and the excitement of the hospice idea. When such zeal is combined with small size and great interdependence of hospice staff, the selection of the right staff for the hospice program becomes very important.

Effective staff development begins before the hiring and is established in the written philosophy and program as well as in the personnel codes and practices of the hospice. The preparation of these important documents should be completed early in the organizational development by the governing board and executive director. These policies should be the outgrowth of the shared expectations of the developers of the program and, although fixed at any moment, should always be subject to revision as new people accumulate new experiences.

The following is a statement of goals and principles developed by Hospice, Inc., of New Haven, Connecticut.

### Goals and Principles

The goals of the Hospice Home Care program are as follows:

1. To ease the overall stress and burden of a traumatic life experience by sharing and working with the expressed needs—physical, emotional, social, and spiritual—of the cancer patient and the family.
2. To aid the patient in the struggle to maintain independence and to experience death with dignity.
3. To minimize the painful and damaging effects of the family's bereavement.

To strengthen the bond between patients and families in need of comprehensive care, and the caregivers, administrators, and citizens who formulate and provide the appropriate services, the following principles have been developed by Hospice.

1. Comprehensive care requires interdisciplinary expertise and broad utilization of other community services. Furthermore, a constant exposure to terminal situations necessitates much peer support and consultation. For the home care team to provide this care, decision-making must be a team effort. The home care "hierarchy" is therefore decentralized to allow constant interchange of ideas and suggestions, as opposed to more traditional physician-dominated decision-making.
2. Both the home care and the administrative bodies need persons who have had contact with other community health organizations, cancer groups, and so forth to facilitate the complex task of coordinating these many services into a therapeutic milieu suitable to varying patient and family needs.
3. Because dialogue with dying patients has been the real key to redesigning terminal care, the clergy and others who regularly counsel patients have played an important role in hospice.
4. Caregivers with previous experience in terminal settings of any kind are valued for technical expertise while lending a certain perspective and stability to the team.*

* Lack, S. A., Buckingham, R. W.: *The First American Hospice—Three Years of Home Care.* The Connecticut Hospice, New Haven, CT, 1978.

The presence of an identified, clearly stated philosophy of care, supported by the organization and adhered to by all staff, is the essential basis of good staff morale and performance.

While there are no hard and fast rules for staff selection, the pre-employment interview is a most important opportunity for interpreting the hospice program and eliciting responses from the applicant. The applicant should be able to deal with questions that clarify the desire to work in hospice, the ability to care for dying persons, the response to grieving families, and a personal sensitivity to how one deals with stress and makes use of a support community.

Interviews with prospective employees should always be conducted in person so that there are opportunities for both parties to interact and question. After initial screening it would be valuable for the applicant to meet with several employees, volunteers, and family members to get a real sense of the composite team working together. This is important because the employment interview should allow the prospective employee to assess the job opportunity to assure that it meets his expectations. Additionally, this process should initiate the new employee into the expected style of interdisciplinary functions and interpersonal support and sharing. There is no better time than at the interview to introduce these expectations. The employee who would find this environment uncomfortable would be best advised of this early to avoid an uncomfortable work situation. The employee who is looking for this kind of interactive work setting will find the interview process part of a rite of entry, and staff members will find themselves renewing their own commitment as they interpret hospice values to the new employee.

It is extremely hard to suggest specific guidelines that would serve all hospice programs equally well. The applicant should meet the expectations for job performance and be able to work and contribute to the hospice program and to a supportive work community. Some believe that an applicant in bereavement would not make a good employee. But what about the applicant who has never experienced the loss of any close personal relationship? Would that person be most or least desirable? What about the person who experienced multiple losses of friends and relatives? How would this person rate? Obviously this one characteristic alone should not determine suitability for work in hospice. Feifel (1963) postulates that one of the reasons people enter the healing professions "is as an unconscious defense against inordinate anxiety about death—an anxiety that has its roots in childhood." The application of this idea to practice might preclude health professionals working with dying persons if we concluded that all health professionals should have resolved their death anxieties. No applicant for hospice employment will have totally resolved his or her own responses to most aspects of life. The persons hospice wants should demonstrate a balance of the qualities of professional competence, compassion, and empathy and especially the sensitivity to their own feelings and the feelings of other staff members. Whatever tools will help staff learn this about the candidate's qualifications should be appropriately utilized.

In addition to the efforts put into the interviewing process, it is especially important not to deemphasize the value of a probationary period as an opportunity to explore the new staff member's interest and capacity to work in hospice. During the probationary period there should be an intensive staff training program that encourages examination of responses to the dying person which can be most helpful to test the appropriateness of hospice employment. This, coupled with actual work in care of the dying, should provide a real test to determine if expectations have been met.

A job becomes attractive because of social approval of the efforts it demands and because of the importance the job has in the community. Social approval of garbage collectors always increases rapidly after the accumulation of garbage on city streets. Respect for people who do the least desirable work increases when other people consider the option of having personally to carry out the undesirable task.

Taking care of the dying person is a job most people would prefer not to do and for that reason there is measured respect for people who elect to do so. However, because of the crisis or trauma associated with dying, people who care for the dying are seen as being at high risk to experience trauma themselves. They should, therefore, be questioned about their motives for exposing themselves to the unhappiness of the work situation. It may be that the expectation of unhappiness and unusual stress in working with the dying has been based on an encounter with unexpected death, a death considered to reflect on the health care worker's professional competence, or a death that poses conflicts between organizational and human values.

What will be the changed societal expectation of hospice staff when communities begin to see death occurring without pain, without inter-organizational conflict, without being interpreted as a loss of professional competence? When hospice care is recognized for helping people experience a peaceful, appropriate death will the social approval of hospice staff be reduced because death will be seen as less threatening? Or will hospice merely be more respectable because the undesirable aspects of caring for the dying will continue?

It is important to consider hospice staff differently from those working with the dying in hospitals, nursing homes, or other situations. Expectations regarding grief, trauma, burnout, and other staff-related problems will have to be established for hospice staff as a distinct subgroup providing care for the dying.

Staff regularly working with families in distress and witnessing the frequent trauma of death need the ready availability of a supportive staff structure where there is dependability in the presence of other people, in their understanding of the nature of the distress, and in their skill in knowing what is the most helpful response.


## A Coping Mechanism

How will the employee know if he is suited to work with the dying? How can the person learn both to deal with the difficulties of this new relationship and to be helpful to the patient?

Harper (1977) has conceptualized a helping framework for the employee who experiences the trauma, pain, and uncertainty encountered by one new to working with death. The Harper paradigm begins with the premise that the new employee is ill-prepared for encounters with death by either his personal background or professional training and will not know how to deal with the uncertainties and anxieties that must be confronted. This requires an adjustment period: a time for reflection, feeling, and working through feelings about this new role. Such a process enables the worker to gain the knowledge and strength necessary to direct his energies into a "new human caring dimension" (Harper, 1977).

The paradigm is organized into a process of time and growth and is illustrated in five stages, requiring approximately twenty-four months to complete. This schema, shown in Figure 5–1, is titled "Coping with Professional Anxiety in Terminal Illness," and the growth sequence is referred to as the "line of comfort-ability."

Harper (1977) developed this paradigm for professionals working with the dying because: "professionals . . . do not enter practice academically, intellectually or emotionally prepared to deal with death and dying. They must learn to cope with professional anxieties arising from such experiences. This requires an adjustment period for the professional, a time for working through his own feelings about death, dying and life's end."

New employees go through an adaptive process in order to become comfortable. It therefore is helpful to identify the process so that it can be taught and then used.

The worker gains understanding, knowledge, and strength and works through conflicts, internal and external, thus adding a new human caring dimension to his existing capacity to be helpful—this is the maturing of the health professional.


### STAGE I   KNOWLEDGE AND ANXIETY

This is the initial period of encountering the dying at which workers are anxious to serve, are concerned but uncomfortable. Tangible requests get priority with intellectualization rather than emotionalism dominating

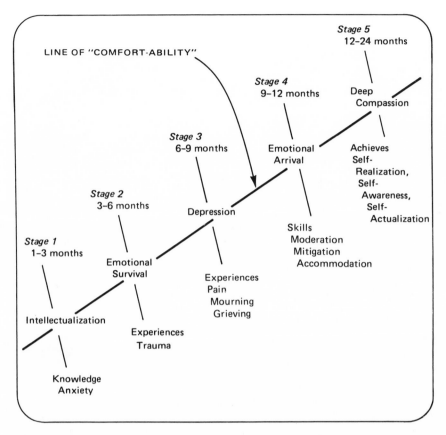

**Figure 5–1**  Coping with Professional Anxiety in Terminal Illness

*Source:* From Bernice Catherine Harper, *Death: The Coping Mechanism of the Health Professional* (Greenville, S.C.: Southeastern University Press, 1977). Reprinted with permission.

the method of handling the problem. The worker is not yet prepared to let the patient talk about death and dying or raise sensitive questions.

### STAGE II  EMOTIONAL SURVIVAL

The worker experiences traumas accompanied by guilt and frustration, and through these feelings confronts the realization of his own eventual death. Guilt and frustration are evoked because the worker lives on in good health and witnesses the deterioration of his patient. The worker realizes the reality of impending death for his patient. Recognizing his inability to arrest the process, he wants to fight back and is jolted out of the inertia of intellectualization into the activity of emotional involvement accompanied by emotional growth.

**Table 5–1**    Stage Characteristics and Differences of the Schematic Growth and Development Scale

| Stage I | Stage II | Stage III | Stage IV | Stage V |
|---------|----------|-----------|----------|---------|
| Professional Knowledge | Increasing Professional Knowledge | Deepening of Professional Knowledge | Acceptance of Professional Knowledge | Refining of Professional Knowledge |
| Intellectualization | Less Intellectualization | Decreasing Intellectualization | Normal Intellectualization | Refining Intellectual Base |
| Anxiety | Emotional Survival | Depression | Emotional Arrival | Deep Compassion |
| Some Uncomfortableness | Increasing Uncomfortableness | Decreasing Uncomfortableness | Increasing Comfortableness | Increased Comfortableness |
| Agreeableness | Guilt | Pain | Moderation | Self-Realization |
| Withdrawal | Frustration | Mourning | Mitigation | Self-Awareness |
| Superficial Acceptance | Sadness | Grieving | Accommodation | Self-Actualization |
| Providing Tangible Services | Initial Emotional Involvement | More Emotional Involvement | Ego Mastery | Professional Satisfaction |
| Utilization of Emotional Energy on Understanding the Setting | Increasing Emotional Involvement | Over-Identification with the Patient | Coping with Loss of Relationship | Acceptance of Death and Loss |
| Familiarizing Self with Policies and Procedures | Initial Understanding of the Magnitude of the Area of Practice | Exploration of Own Feelings about Death | Freedom from Concern about Own Death | Rewarding Professional Growth and Development |
| Working with Families Rather than Patients | Over-Identification with the Patient's Situation | Facing Own Death | Developing Strong Ties with Dying Patients and Families | Development of Ability to Give of One's Self |
| | | Coming to Grips with Feelings about Death | Development of Ability to Work with, on Behalf of and for the Dying Patient | Human and Professional Assessment |
| | | | Development of Professional Competence | Constructive and Appropriate Activities |

**Table 5–1**  *continued*

| Stage I | Stage II | Stage III | Stage IV | Stage V |
|---------|----------|-----------|----------|---------|
| | | | Productivity and Accomplishments | Development of Feelings of Dignity and Self-Respect |
| | | | Healthy Interaction | Ability to Give Dignity and Self-Respect to Dying Patient |
| | | | | Feeling of Comfortableness in Relation to Self, Patient, Family, and the Job |

*Source:* From Bernice Catherine Harper, *Death: The Coping Mechanism of the Health Professional* (Greenville, S.C.: Southeastern University Press, 1977). Reprinted with permission.

STAGE III   DEPRESSION

In this stage the worker experiences extreme anxiety, grief, and depression. Usefulness and capability are questioned. This stage is referred to as the "grow or go" stage because if the frustrations and pain are too great or are not adequately rewarded, if grieving and mourning are overwhelming and the worker cannot "grow" in personal strength and capacity, it is better for the worker to "go." The worker who goes on at this point without the growth will unquestionably die a million deaths.

If at this time the question, "Isn't working with dying persons depressing?" is frequently encountered, it must be answered strongly in the negative by the worker who is to survive. The worker at this stage should be concerned by the dilemma of the person dying who lacks appropriate responses from the health care providers, or the inappropriate way in which the person is dying.

STAGE IV   EMOTIONAL ARRIVAL

This stage is marked by a sense of freedom from the debilitating effects of the pain and grief. The worker has the resilience to recover and has the control to practice his art.

The worker is freed from identifying with symptoms and with guilt and is no longer preoccupied with his own death. Instead, sensitivities have increased and, while not free from pain, he is free from its incapacitating effects.

### Stage V  Deep Compassion

This stage is characterized by self-realization, self-awareness, and self-actualization and is the culmination of all of the growth and development that has previously transpired. The worker has the willingness and capacity to serve the dying, coupled with a feeling of his own worth that communicates comfort and respect to the dying person.

This systemization of the coping mechanism for working with dying persons has implications for staff development. As for other stage theories, the usual admonitions should be posited to avoid the requirement that every staff member conform to the same sequencing, time frame, and ultimate product. The schema is valuable, nonetheless, offering a goal for workers' greater self-awareness and a goal-oriented sequence of events. Furthermore, it helps the worker leaving the cycle find the best time to jump off. All health workers need not work with dying persons. It is to be hoped that all will deal with their own mortality and, therefore, deliberate on the meaning of their own lives. This process should make them more effective practitioners of interpersonal relationships because of their ability to respond to the needs of the patient and be comfortable with their own role.

## Staff Development

A well-designed, helpful orientation program is a requirement for all new employees. It should also serve as an introduction to an ongoing program of continuing education for all hospice staff. The following is an illustration of objectives for a staff training program.

### Objectives

The program should be designed so that each staff member:

1. Knows the philosophy of caring for patients in hospice.
2. Learns about the expectations of patient's needs during the last period of life and the responses made available through the hospice program.
3. Learns about the specific progression of cancer and the expectations for care in the terminal stages of the illness.
4. Becomes more aware of his own feelings about death and is, thereby, more comfortable with them.

5. Becomes familiar with the different religious and cultural practices and beliefs related to death and dying.
6. Is introduced to the concept of team functioning and learns communication strategies and skills.
7. Learns about bereavement, grieving, and mourning and the hospice role with survivors.
8. Understands the health and social care delivery systems and their resources for hospice.
9. Understands the organization policies and practices related to employment.

Hillhaven Hospice, Tucson, Arizona, has designed a framework for staff development based on a progression of skills, methods of instruction, and evaluation procedures. This is shown in Figure 5–2 with a description of the content. It is introduced by forty hours of orientation provided during the first week of employment. This is followed by ongoing educational sessions, participation in the staff support community, and self-paced learning based on each employee's needs for additional content information. An important part of the orientation week is devoted to experiential self-awareness activities designed to help the employee direct his thoughts to the issues related to the meaning of life, dying, death, and caring for the dying person. A series of exercises has been developed to assist the new employee to look at his own experience in dealing with death. "The full preciousness and uniqueness of life becomes fully available to us only when we understand that death is personal and not just for others" (Feifel, 1977). If death were less a stranger to us we could live with the concept as a realistic backdrop that accentuates the importance of life and its experiences (Feifel, 1977).

The exercises are introduced by the use of the "Hospice Discussion Guide," shown in Table 5–2, which provides the opportunity for personal introductions and sharing values about dying and death. The group is organized in pairs who spend about five minutes getting to know something about one another. The "Hospice Discussion Guide" is then distributed with instructions that the pairs be retained and continue to discuss each of the questions thoroughly. There is no interest in consensus. The point is in having each person explore his own values and solicit the expression of the partner's values. After thirty to forty minutes of this exchange, individuals are invited to comment on their disagreements or agreements with any of the issues discussed or to raise questions about any of the statements in the discussion guide. The group members are usually well prepared to defend some of their own positions during this open discussion. The goal of the discussion is to show that there is generally a wide range of different feelings expressed about most of the topics introduced in the discussion guide.

**Figure 5–2** Framework for Staff Development Program

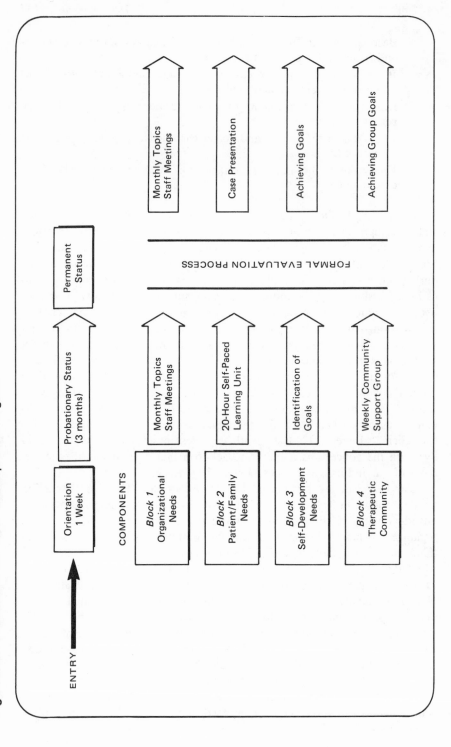

## Block 1—ORGANIZATIONAL NEEDS

*Orientation*

To Hillhaven Foundation
To Hillhaven Hospice
To personnel policies
To policies and procedures
To position description
To patient's rights
To personnel

*Ongoing*

Timely implementation/review of operational guidelines

## Block 2—PATIENT/FAMILY NEEDS

*Orientation*

Communication skills
Needs of dying patients/families
Hospice model of pain control
Patient care conferences
Symptom control

*First Three Months*

Basic counseling skills
Nature of pain
Needs of the older person
Legal/ethical issues
Family dynamics
Transcultural care
Behavioral responses to illness
Loss and grief

*Ongoing*

Biology of cancer
Pharmacology
Organic brain syndrome
Functional confusion
Treatment modalities
Comparative religions
Reality orientation
Home care
Discharge counseling
Family education
Bereavement

## Block 3—SELF-DEVELOPMENT NEEDS

*Orientation*

Team membership
Group process
Conference skills
Interpersonal relationships
Experimental self-awareness activities
Burnout/stress reduction
Death anxiety
Physical fitness program

*First Three Months*

Identification/setting self goals
Group membership
Committee work
Patient/family case presentation
Resources for self care

*Permanent Status*

Achieving self goals
Dealing with stress

## Block 4—THERAPEUTIC COMMUNITY

*Orientation*

Community support group
Multidisciplinary team
Group awareness
Group goals

*Ongoing*

Achieving group goals

## End of Three Months — FORMAL EVALUATION PROCESS

*By Supervisor/Peers*

Hospice concept
Position evaluation
Knowledge/implementation of policies and procedures
Knowledge and skill application

*Of Self*

Death anxiety
Stress reduction
Goal setting/achieving
"Fit" into community

*Orientation Program by Employee*

Orientation program
Learning modules

*Source:* From Hillhaven Hospice, Tucson, Arizona. Reprinted with permission.

**Table 5–2**  Hospice Discussion Guide

These questions are provided to stimulate discussion. While there are no "correct" responses, the questionnaire is intended to elicit your opinion.

1. Nurses do not like to talk about death.
2. Everybody fears death.
3. Patients should be allowed to die without resuscitation measures.
4. A nurse should not become too involved with dying patients so that she can function efficiently.
5. People shouldn't have to die alone.
6. Every patient has a right to know that he is dying.
7. Care staff should be consistent in approaches to the dying patient.
8. Euthanasia is appropriate under certain circumstances.
9. My first experience with death was (will be) very painful.
10. Patients should be allowed to go through the stages of death.
11. Care of the terminally ill can best be provided at home.
12. Death is an end to suffering.
13. I feel guilty when patients die.
14. Care providers should let patients introduce the topic of death.
15. Life-saving measures should be interrupted at the discretion of the physician.
16. All suffering has meaning.
17. Hospice care is the same as long-term care in a nursing home.
18. "Modern medicine is devoted to the preservation of life, and death is viewed as an intrusion into a scientific quest for eternal existence."
19. Touch is very important to the dying patient.
20. I fear death.
21. Care providers should not allow patients and families to see them cry.
22. Life exists after death in another form.
23. Part of the fear of dying is fear of loss of self-control.
24. Doctors feel uncomfortable talking about death.
25. Man has the right to die with dignity.
26. Control of symptoms is the physician's responsibility.
27. Counseling is part of each staff person's responsibility in hospice care.
28. Hospice care is comparable to euthanasia.

This exercise is then followed by drawings of death on a large sheet of newsprint (27 by 32 inches). Each person is asked to draw his or her impression of death. It is helpful if colored crayons are available for the drawings. Participants should be advised that they will be invited to share their drawings with the entire group but that they may elect not to do so. Those who wish to share are then asked to describe their drawings and personal interpretations of death. Each participant is given the opportunity to interpret, to himself and others, his own feelings about death. The others have their perspective broadened as they have the opportunity to hear their co-workers' reactions to death.

The session can end with a discussion of recollections of participants' first encounters with death and the meaning this had for them. If the group has more than six to eight persons, there probably will not be time for this third exercise during a two-hour period. It is important that each participant know that the group leader will be available for personal follow-up on any issues raised as a result of these discussions and that a follow-up session with the entire group will be scheduled within a few days.

The second session should be dedicated to a follow-up of the discussions in the first session with attention given to the expression of the feelings of each of the participants. The participants are then urged to read *New Meanings of Death* by Feifel (1977), and the group continues to meet, discussing issues in the readings or work experiences. After one month, the focus of the group should be changed to emphasize the meaning of "community" as the support group in hospice. New employees are integrated into the existing meeting schedules when they complete this part of the orientation.

## Developing a Caring Community

How does the hospice team become a community? What is a working hospice community and how does it differ from the team? While the team and community both work together for some common goal or purpose, the community has relationships that exceed the expectations of a multidisciplinary team.

**Principle:** *A caring community must develop from the team of caregivers, not only to collaborate in providing patient care, but also to offer support to one another. The caring community requires a strong bond evolving from mutual regard and interpersonal involvement. Community members not only share and work together, but also recognize that individual capacity to function depends upon the wholeness and relatedness of all team members. The group becomes a community when each member is committed to the other members and all community members feel and know intense interpersonal commitment.*

**Discussion:** Community support gives members strength to reach out comfortably to a member of the team in distress. Team members know when one of them is overwhelmed and needs relief and should then encourage the team member to withdraw temporarily. Such withdrawal is perceived not as failure but as a need for rest while others in the community pick up the slack. Interpersonal attachments bind hospice workers together as they deal with death and loss.

The sense of community does not necessarily evolve on its own, although that may occur when there is strong leadership and commitment.

Sometimes it may be difficult to assign responsibilities for the development of community to any one staff person or discipline because leadership depends on a person, not a position. Who should be assigned the leadership role for the community? It will vary with the composition of the staff, their interests and strengths. In any case, one or more staff members should be made responsible for the development of community. It should be noted that purposeful staff involvement in the development of a sense of community may be related to in-service education but may not necessarily be the same thing. Skills required to develop a sense of community differ from those needed to teach a caring function. It would be a mistake to limit responsibility for developing a sense of community to the staff person responsible for staff education. Developing community is a group responsibility, even an expectation of all members of the staff. Community develops out of the successful management of team stress and conflict. Conflict is unavoidable and must be appreciated as an expected occurrence in interpersonal relationships. Rather than permitting conflict to make a group dysfunctional, its power should be understood and managed to strengthen the interrelationships among members of the staff.

Appreciation of the differences between staff education and staff development sets the stage for development of understanding of the multiple levels of staff training required by a hospice program. At one level, staff members must be made aware of the philosophy and goals of the organization and of all its peripheral concerns. These will include personnel and payroll, fire safety and emergency procedures, and control of infection. Depending upon individual background and education, training in patient care, with emphasis on care of dying persons, will be another level of education. Time must be devoted to the ideas, values, and expectations of hospice. The license category of hospice may very well carry with it expectations for certain levels of staff education, therefore programs may vary depending upon the expressed expectations of the regulations.

At yet another level, every new hospice employee must be encouraged to benefit from increased sensitivity to the needs of the dying person and his family. Such sensitivity can be enhanced by experiential exercises in the meaning of death and loss. While exercises and the styles of presenters will differ, it is important that staff be helped to examine their own feelings about death and to explore their own encounters with death and loss. The orientation program is, in fact, the beginning of community as participants begin to share and sense support from other staff members, as well as to appreciate the importance of staff supports.

After orientation, it is important that new employees be integrated into the existing staff community to facilitate their feelings of inclusion in the organization.

Development of community is closely related to staff development.

Typically there are four levels of staff meetings as part of staff development. Each function of staff meetings has different goals. These include:

1. In-service education programs intended to enhance each person's skill level in dealing with care responsibilities. Such issues as behavioral problems, family relations, drug interactions, and pain control are illustrative of appropriate topics. The staff development person will generally prepare material for these educational meetings based on the staff needs.
2. Regular case management meetings at which staff members review the care program and progress of each hospice participant and his or her family. These reviews serve the educational objectives of improving care through the examination and assessment of current practices and are coordinated by the medical director. They should be held frequently.
3. Staff members should be involved in administrative meetings focused on aspects of management of hospice. The greater the involvement of staff in significant decisions, the greater will be their involvement in goals of the organization as a whole. The quality of the caring community is enhanced when all staff members are aware of the many administrative problems involved in organizing, funding, and directing a hospice program and can join together to help solve some of the problems. These meetings are coordinated by the executive director.
4. Community meetings offer opportunities for building staff supports, understanding areas of problems in personal interrelationships, and strengthening team functioning. These meetings should be coordinated by the person responsible for developing the community, who may be the social worker, psychiatrist, or other staff person with skills in group interaction and development.

## Burnout

Each staff member, and especially the administrator, should be sensitive to evidence of staff hostility, anger, withdrawal, or other symptoms that might suggest either a breakdown in the community or the inability of some staff members to function in hospice. These symptoms may be evidence of "burnout," the inability to handle the intensity of the hospice environment, and may call for immediate intervention to respond appropriately to the staff member's needs.

Burnout has been defined by Pines and Maslack (1978) as "a syndrome of physical and emotional exhaustion, involving the development of negative self-concept, negative job analysis, and loss of concern and feeling for clients." Burnout seems to occur for health care providers as a result of continued interpersonal interventions in the lives of people in distress. The problems seem to be exacerbated when the patient-staff ratio is so high as to cause the staff to feel out of control, or unable to relate comfortably to each of the patients (Maslack, 1976). This ratio would obviously vary with the capacities of each staff person as well as the needs and problems of each patient. This means that a work assignment schedule should consider patient needs and the demand load on the person rather than simply numbers of patients or staff members.

"Opportunities for withdrawal from a stressful situation are critically important" (Maslack, 1976), and providing "times out" in the sense of short breaks, days off, and variation in job assignments seems to be an effective method to avoid burnout.

"To combat burnout from intense work with clients, staff in the human services use such techniques as detached concern, intellectualization, withdrawal from clients, and sharp separation of work from home life" (Pines and Maslack, 1978). These become the defensive tools of the individual attempting to cope with the personal distress. Obviously these manifestations are counterproductive to the close involvement hospice staff need to have with their patients but are important tools for the self-preservation of the staff person. Oftentimes burnout leads to a deterioration of physical health and may be manifested in illness, absenteeism, or increased use of alcohol and drugs.

Staff stress can be reduced by varying work tasks. For example, staff can be utilized for community education programs or to provide orientation and tours for visitors. Having flexible scheduling for time off permits staff to respond to their own perceived stress and enables them to request time off as needed.

Because concerns for staff burnout should always be present, hospice programs must pursue a positive course of action to respond to staff needs and to avoid the painful distress of burnout and its ultimate negative impact on patient care.

A positive program to offset burnout is in fact analogous to a standard personnel program appropriate for hospice. When stress and grief can be anticipated because of the nature of the role of hospice, much can be done to avoid the deleterious impact on staff and patients. This does not mean to expect a reduction of standards of performance or expectations from hospice personnel. It merely advocates for those positive actions that could be interpreted to represent sound occupational health and safety.

The following should be expected as part of the hospice personnel program.

1. The program should begin with the assumption that the hospice environment, although related to dying, death, and grief, will be less stressful than the more traditional health care environments

where death is confronted. This is so because of the reduction of staff and organizational conflict between the need to sustain life and the desire to help achieve an appropriate death. Hospice is committed to the appropriate death so staff can be relieved of this source of stress.

2. The prospective employee is introduced to hospice with a clear statement of the philosophy and program.
3. Positive community regard for hospice bestows a social approval and value on the service that contributes to the importance of each employee's participation.
4. An in-person interview, especially with members of the team and patients, clearly introduces the working environment and identifies expectations for the prospective employee.
5. A probationary period providing a transitional time for self-explorations and better understanding of the environment is important.
6. Formulating a framework for coping with the personal expectations of working in a hospice program is helpful to new staff as a guideline for expected growth and increased competence. The framework developed by Harper (1977), titled "Coping with Professional Anxiety in Terminal Illness," as described in Figure 5–1, is one suggested approach.
7. A well-designed orientation program completed prior to beginning clinical practice should be available in addition to an ongoing continuing education program. The orientation should include experiential exercises designed to increase the employee's sensitivities to the many issues that will be confronted in dealing with death.
8. Work assignments should permit the employee to carry out the caring expected in the hospice program.
9. Work relief and rotation should contribute to staff refreshment and renewal.
10. Regular participation in a staff support system meeting emphasizes interpersonal sharing, as does sharing in hospice-sponsored social activities.

## Multidisciplinary Team

The ability to implement a hospice program is, for the most part, a reflection of the capacity of staff, both individually and as a group. The issues related to selection, training, assignment, and staff supports must be foremost in the design of a hospice program. The varied professional disciplines that relate to the quality of life in health care, together with volunteers make up a multidisciplinary staff. The hospice team must be a community of caring to be effective—caring for patients, their families, staff, and themselves. The individuals selected for hospice work have a special opportunity to demonstrate humane care of dying persons, including providing staff support.

**Principle:** *The staff of a hospice is a multidisciplinary team that makes up a caring, competent, and therapeutic community. Under the overall direction of an administrator and the medical direction of a physician, its members should include nurses, social workers, physical and occupational therapists, chaplain, clinical pharmacologist, activity workers, and case manager. Volunteers comprise an integral part of the team of caregivers. At the minimum the team includes the patient and a significant other person.*

**Discussion:**    While individuals make up a team, the hospice care team is more than a collection of individuals. It is its individual members, plus the philosophy of hospice care, plus the commitment of each person, plus the dying person and family and, finally, the caring community. The caring community is essentially the goal of staff development, for it is through that support structure that hospice care is provided. The unusual nature of the concentrated care of dying persons and their families requires a strong team approach, both for those who receive care and those providing care. The importance of staff support and the role of the team in providing support must be stressed at the outset. The care provided by the team is good for the person receiving care if it also provides for the staff's needs, morale, and ability to function at a highly effective level. Staff members must be understood, supported, and recognized positively for their caring. While there are hierarchical differences within the team, defined by position and title, or education, or length of employment, there is no point in artificially denying these differences. No team member should be denied his or her legitimate role on the team; appropriate carrying out of that role should be acknowledged. Roles need not be static and positions in the team structure can change because people grow in their social functioning, personal strength, and professional skills. Such growth should both be fostered by changing expectations from the team and rewarded by the team and hospice administration.

The team composition is important because care is not being provided to an organ or illness but to a living individual who is involved in a social network. Multiple needs cannot adequately be met by caregivers of any single discipline. The dying person and family need options, and they must be able to choose relationships with members of the team whom they perceive as being best able to meet their needs. The team concept also is important because it provides staff members the internal support they need to become a caring community.

All who participate in the care must be part of the team. Many times

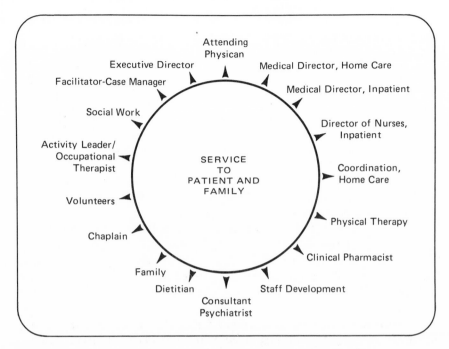

**Figure 5–3** Staff Components of Hospice Caring Community

*Source:* Adapted from Dr. William Farr, Medical Director, Hillhaven Hospice, Tucson, Arizona. Reprinted with permission.

roles will overlap and in some situations roles may be interchangeable. The needs of the dying person dictate how each team member functions (Lamerton, 1973).

TEAM MEMBERS

The *administrator* of hospice is the manager and coordinator of the overall program, overseeing the entire operation, dealing with human services, and making their delivery possible. The administrator is frequently the person who interprets a hospice program to the community, represents the service among other health care agencies, and provides liaison with the governing board.

The administrator should have appropriate training and experience in the management of health care services and should be experienced in working with health care providers and community service agencies. No complex health care program can exist without coordination of funding resources, and it is especially important that the administrator be skilled in this area.

The *physician* is the key person directing the care of the dying person.

Medical care continues whether the goal is cure or comfort. The doctor must prescribe drugs for management of pain and alleviation of nausea as well as treatments or comfort measures for management of incontinence and/or constipation. The physician is the professional director of hospice medical care and its most important liaison with the medical community. The attending physician should continue to provide the primary medical care and as such should be a member of the team planning for his patient. Community physicians will sometimes refer patients to the hospice medical director for assistance with pain or other symptom control.

The hospice physician refers patients to other medical resources such as radiation therapy as an adjunct in pain relief. Physician management makes it possible for hospice patients to move back into the acute care system when such a referral is deemed appropriate.

The *facilitator* is the liaison person between hospice and community and manager of the patient in the hospice system. Hospice care of the patient and family begins with the facilitator as an intake worker. It is recommended that this person be a registered nurse with a strong background in both nursing and counseling. The facilitator assesses all patients referred to hospice prior to admission and will visit with the applicant at home or in the hospital and arrange for a visit to the inpatient facility when appropriate. In consultation with the attending physician, family, and other team members, the facilitator recommends the level of care most appropriate, i.e., home care, inpatient care, etc., and arranges for those services to be offered. These plans must be arranged in a very short time period, often on the same day as the request for service is made.

The facilitator has a key role, serving as advocate for the patient and family as long as the service is provided.

Following the death of a patient, the facilitator activates the system of continued assistance to provide comfort, guidance, and information to the family during bereavement.

The *nurse* provides the primary care supporting the patient's ability to live as fully as possible within the limitations imposed by illness. Nurses care for patients on a twenty-four-hour basis in the inpatient unit and deal with their physical care and their psychosocial needs. The nurse is the professional most readily available to those in the inpatient facility. For home-care patients, it is the nurse who works with the patient, teaches the family, and is probably the most frequently seen member of the hospice team. Giving a bath or helping the patient move about brings the nurse into close physical contact with the patient, promoting communication opportunities. It is the nurse who provides information, explanations, and instructions. While in intimate contact with the patient, the nurse has opportunities for family contact and exchange.

Nurses, then, can share their knowledge of each patient, their assessments of patient needs, their definitions of problems, and their evaluations of results with the care team as a whole. A multifaceted perspective is then achieved, with the nurses' input as a valuable component.

The director of nursing coordinates inpatient nursing care services, and the home-care coordinator provides the same services for home care.

A nursing staff will generally consist of registered nurses, licensed practical nurses, and nursing assistants.

The *chaplain* brings another perspective to the care of dying patients—the meeting of spiritual needs. The chaplain provides opportunities for individual religious expression related to the needs of the patient and the family unit. The hospice chaplain must not be a provider or promoter of any single religion or religious practice, however. He provides a link to the religious community for patients and for the staff. The chaplain has a critical function of helping the patient's own clergy be more knowledgeable and effective. The hospice respects the right of each person to worship or not to worship. Those with no religious affiliation, and those with special beliefs, must be assured that their desires will be respected. Some patients and/or family members will choose the chaplain as the person with whom they can communicate and find comfort. A nondenominational chapel in the inpatient unit should be available for use by patients, family, and friends unless the hospice is sponsored by a religious group. The chaplain may sometimes lead services; sometimes other clergy from the community may be invited to do so. The hospice chaplain participates as a team member in helping whoever may be involved understand religious practices as they are related to patients whether in home care or inpatient care. In addition, he may explain religious practices, assisting staff in their understanding of patients and patient needs. The chaplain should be an important member of the bereavement team.

The *social worker* should be professionally trained and preferably be a person with a master's degree in social work. The social worker is concerned with the adaptive potential of people and the supportive qualities of their environment and strives to improve the transaction between the patient and his environment in order to enhance the adaptive capacities. In addition to providing services to the patient, to the patient and family, and to family members and staff, the social worker should serve as a member of the bereavement team.

The *physical therapist* has as a goal to help plan activity that will maximize the patient's diminishing resources, rather than to improve function. The physical therapist should be involved in both the home-care program and the inpatient facility, teaching the family to assist the patient with necessary or desirable activities such as moving from bed to chair.

The *activities leader* may be an occupational therapist or a recreation therapist. The level of activity at which an individual patient will participate is very much dependent upon current physical condition and ability as well as desire to be active. The activity director plans social activities such as parties and picnics as well as devising work programs for individual patients either at home or in the inpatient facility.

An important contribution of the activity program should be provision of opportunities for self-expression and creativity. Many of the hospice activities will be with individuals or family units rather than with groups of patients. The focus on activities may help family members find a more comfortable way to relate to the dying person without focusing on the dying experience. Creative activities may provide an outlet for some patients and families to be expressive about their dealing with dying.

The *staff development* person has overall responsibility for the process that attracts new staff to hospice, oversees the orientation and training of the total staff, and assures that appropriate leadership is provided to the staff community. This person should see that appropriate measures are instituted to avoid burnout and should encourage staff socialization through extracurricular picnics, parties, etc. Appropriate studies should be conducted to understand problems of staff turnover and measures taken to respond appropriately to these problems.

A *consultant psychiatrist* should be available to assist staff members in their dealing with difficult personal or family situations encountered in hospice care. The psychiatrist should be an important resource to the staff community by either providing leadership or by assisting other staff in this leadership.

The psychiatrist may also contribute to diagnosis of problems and development of treatment plans as part of the multidisciplinary staff.

The *dietitian* must respond to the special dietary needs of the patient and family, assuring that individual needs, and especially preferences, are met. The unique eating schedules and problems people may have with eating have to be accounted for in developing the dietary program.

The *clinical pharmacist* coordinates and supervises pharmaceutical services for inpatients and home-care patients. The drugs the patient receives are monitored, and the pharmacist educates patients and their families regarding medication. Hospice nursing staff members can consult with the pharmacist regarding clients' drugs and their interactions. The clinical pharmacist is the expert consultant to hospice physicians on reactions to drugs. Together with nurses and medical staff, the pharmacist monitors and evaluates patient responses.

*Volunteers* are very much part of a hospice program. They can act as activity assistants, help with inpatient care, assist with clerical work and receptions, transport patients, and help with small chores such as providing reading material. Volunteers link the community to the hospice facility and can also act as "friendly visitors" to home-care patients, provide constant companionship to the dying person, and provide bereavement services.

The nature of hospice service makes volunteers important members of the care team. Volunteers provide a variety of services, based on individual capacity and skills. The volunteer should never be considered a second-rate staff person; the recruitment, screening, training, and supervision of volunteers should be comparable to that provided for paid employees. Volunteers should be included in staff and community meetings, and they should participate when appropriate in team meetings and other educational sessions. Expectations of volunteers must be high, and each individual volunteer must be given enough training and involvement to help assure successful performance.

Not all volunteers are skilled in interpersonal relations with dying persons or comfortable with them. Some may be very skilled in this area. Volunteers who so prefer can be used in a variety of roles covering all the management and service aspects of the hospice community.

The *family* is definitely part of the care team. An important goal of hospice is to strengthen and maintain family ties. Family members may be involved in giving care both at home and in hospice, whenever it seems appropriate. The interdisciplinary team functions *with* as well as *on behalf of* the patient and his family; patient and family should have input into decisions regarding care to be given as well as being recipients of care. Nursing staff should be prepared to instruct family in caring procedures through individual or group sessions. Nursing staff has the main liaison function between hospice care and the family.

To help hospice staff members function in an integrated hospice program, it is desirable for every staff member to rotate through the inpatient and home-care programs in order to have a sense of identity with the entire program. Some staff may be enabled to rotate work assignments, providing a variety of experiences. This, for some persons, may also offset the trauma of repeating the same assignments on a regular basis.

## Summary

Working in a context of frequent exposure to death can be emotionally taxing to staff. How can staff be expected to deal with the intimate experience of death without demonstrating a strong and emotional response? Hospice, because of its acceptance of death, is a program that enables staff to be most responsive to the needs of the dying person. Community acceptance of hospice has brought a new regard for hospice staff and greater acceptance of the caring role for dying persons. Yet in spite of these advances, hospice staff must be carefully selected, oriented, trained, and supported in order to provide the specialized care that characterizes hospice. Ultimately, hospice care will be only as good as the staff supplies, so staff members must have the understanding, organization, and supports necessary to enable them to provide a nurturing, caring environment.

# 6

## The Hospice Environment

*The prime goal of Hospice is to enable both patient
and family to live effectively in the face of impending
death. How can a building help do this?*

Lo-Yi Chan

*We need a sense of institutions. We'll always need some
health care factories for efficient, short term intensive care
stays, but we'll need others where humanity won't
have to overcome the technical apparatus.*

John Thompson and Grace Gold

*But there's one thing you must do: Create a place
of beauty. Even for the dying, beauty is healing.*

Lo-Yi Chan

CREATING A SENSE of beauty is what we should strive for in creating institutional environments. We should accept also that there is beauty in each person's home if it provides the comforts and security the resident requires. It would also be fair to say that no beauty in the environment can substitute for the essential characteristics of staff, program, and caring that should be part of hospice. Beauty, then, is the compatible relationship between the staff and an environment that supports and assists that staff in reaching the goals that comprise total care. The environment should be the outgrowth of those goals in its contribution to the overall mission of hospice.

## Importance of Environment

Thompson and Goldin (1975) describe the design of any nursing unit as composed of four ingredients:

The healthful environment it provides for patients.
The amount of privacy it allows patients.
The extent to which it exercises supervision and control over patients.
The efficiency with which it can be operated.

Noting that these four ingredients are closely interrelated, these writers point out that any variable in one ingredient will have immediate impact on the other three. Similar criteria hold true for the hospice setting, but hospice seeks a different balance, placing special emphasis on individualized care and privacy. These are the characteristics most important to staff members' ability to perform their function of care of the terminally ill. In hospice less importance is placed on the clinical competence for diagnostic procedures or life-saving techniques. Instead the emphasis is on life-preserving qualities enabling family and patient to use their remaining time together most comfortably. Efficiency and patient control in this style are less significant than in curing or rehabilitative settings. Obviously, this is not a plea for inefficiency or poor care, but where a system can at best be less than perfect, a tilt in the direction of personal comforts and privacy is the direction hospice should favor.

In no way should privacy be confused with isolation. Privacy can be achieved in the midst of others if there is the ability to control the environment to suit changing personal needs, accommodate visitors, or provide periods when the individual can be alone.

Privacy can also be aided or adversely affected by the scale and size of the institutional environment. A sense of bigness can be felt in a small environment, and intimacy can be achieved in large institutions. Because hospice programs should primarily support home care, the size of the institutional setting should be small as well as intimate.

It is also important that the hospice environment add to the list of ingredients of the nursing unit a willingness to permit the patient to control his own environment. This may require flexibility of room arrangements, location of bed, extent of privacy or exposure to nurses, and ability to accommodate family members without difficulty.

Most of the comments in this chapter will be directed to readers interested in the design of institutional environments.

Architectural modification or redesign of the home of a person in the final stage of cancer usually is not practical. Some accommodations, such as the use of a hospital bed or safety side rails, may be required to assist the caregivers and protect the patient. A bedside commode may be needed if a toilet is not immediately accessible; an overbed table or bedside table may make the telephone, meals, and toilet articles more accessible. A bedside call bell provides a sense of security when helpers are out of immediate reach but within the household. In some homes the bed might be relocated to the living room so that a sense of isolation or distance is removed. A room with a large sliding door to a patio might make a comfortable bedroom, permitting the patient to get a full view of the garden and the outdoors. Other devices that make a patient comfortable at home should be considered. The goal should be to remove physical restrictions and provide as much patient self-sufficiency as possible. A nurse who has public health experience may be an excellent resource person for help in adapting the home environment to meet the needs of a family that includes a person who is terminally ill. Hospice home-care staff should be prepared to offer appropriate suggestions for minor alterations of furniture or location of bed, or additional appliances that would be useful. After minor modifications of the environment, attention should be directed to the patient.

Literature or research on institutional design specifically tailored for a hospice program is significantly unavailable. Some research is currently in progress at Hillhaven Hospice, Tucson, Arizona, where a postoccupancy evaluation of a hospice building is being conducted. Some generalizations can be gleaned from other institutional designs, however, and should be considered as they relate to modifications of existing buildings or construction of facilities to meet the special needs of the terminally ill.

**Principle:**    *Hospice design should 1) stress homelike characteristics and provide a living environment, 2) recognize the low energy level of its residents, 3) reflect the involvement of family members, 4) provide for patient privacy, 5) offer staff convenience, and 6) allow patient control of the environment.*

**Discussion:**    An initial assumption is made that the person using the institutional environment will be depleted of energy and unable to move about independently. Additionally, there is the assumption that many family members will be present, not merely to observe or visit, but to be active participants in providing care. The hospice environment should provide for continuing living experiences; therefore social spaces, lounges, dining areas, chapel, and recreation rooms should be included and be readily accessible to the patients. All door openings should be wide enough to permit beds to pass through them, and social spaces should be large enough to accommodate several beds.

Why do people enter the inpatient facility if the main thrust of hospice is to provide care at home? First, there are times when the family cannot continue to provide care, where respite is needed or where family is not present and available. The continuity of management, staff, and hospice practices makes it easier on the patient and family to utilize the inpatient unit rather than explore a new institution.

A second reason also is advanced for having an inpatient facility. In the home setting, the patient and family may become socially isolated and come to prefer the ongoing supports of an institutional environment at this time of heightened stress. In the inpatient unit, the presence of volunteers, staff, other patients, and families makes contact with other people easily accessible. An environment which facilitates this contact, while allowing privacy when privacy is desired, is a key to the successful inpatient unit.

Not only does the inpatient unit provide the opportunity for contact with people outside the family, it also provides the opportunity for contact with people experiencing a similar crisis. Very deep friendships are possible between family members and between patients. These associations offer the opportunity to learn from another family just a step ahead on the journey, the opportunity to share experiences with other people experiencing the same crisis, and the opportunity to guide and encourage people who have yet to face what one has just experienced. All this becomes possible when several families are brought together because their members are in the inpatient facility. In addition, whether or not families become friends, there can be tremendous relief and reassurance in seeing death handled as a normal, sad, but not traumatic event. The patient sees that life does go on even after one person's death. The family sees that the patient will be comfortable, not be left alone unwillingly, and that comfort and aid will be available at all times. Sadness, grief, despair, crying, tears, prayer, smiles, and loving comfort will all be observed by families and patients in hospice whenever a patient dies. But these are things that are manageable, survivable. The paralyzing fear of pain, the terror of the unknown, are assuaged by seeing the deaths of others treated as normal events of life.

It should be possible to provide some of these benefits to families at home, and this can be done through the support of volunteers and by including home-care patients and families in the scheduled events at the inpatient facility. This would be especially true of the family program.

### PATIENT'S BEDROOM

One of the most important areas is the inpatient's bedroom, and special attention must be given to the size, number of beds, and furnishings of that room. The most crucial, and as yet unresolved, question in the planning of the patient's bedroom is the number of occupants per room. In English hospices, wards of four beds are common. Several advantages are claimed for this set-up. Since one of the fears of many dying persons is abandonment, the ward arrangement provides constant companionship of other people. Each patient can interact with several other patients as well as have increased contact with staff and visitors. When a nurse or visitor comes to see one patient, each of the other patients in the ward will also receive at least a greeting and polite inquiry, if not more extensive attention. In addition, each patient will probably have the opportunity to watch another patient die. This is an effective rehearsal for one's own death and may alleviate a patient's anxiety about his own death.

Lo-Yi Chan, the architect of the building used by the Connecticut hospice, was profoundly influenced in his choice of a four-bed ward by the experience of the English hospices. Yet it is debatable whether the four-bed ward concept is appropriate to the particular needs of American patients. Americans are used to more privacy, larger homes, separate bedrooms. American hospitals provide private or semiprivate rooms. English hospitals provide large wards. An English patient moving from an eight-person hospital ward to a four-person hospice ward is gaining privacy. An American moving from a private hospital room to a four-bed hospice ward may be losing privacy.

Research in American psychiatric hospitals suggests that providing patients with private rooms actually increases their social participation (Ittelson, 1970). If private bedrooms are provided in a setting where there are other spaces for socialization, such as a dayroom, patients can choose when and with whom and where to socialize. They can invite people into their own rooms and have private conversations without fear of disturbing a roommate or of being overheard, or they can move out to the dayroom or parlor or lounge and join whoever and whatever activity may be going on. However, if patients share bedrooms with other patients, they may have to work hard to find the privacy not provided architecturally, and they may do this by isolating themselves in their own bedrooms, cutting off meaningful interaction with other people.

A private room, on the other hand, gives the patient the option of privacy or of seeking company. Because a hospice patient often has very limited mobility, he may not be able to act on a desire to move from his own room to a social area. This problem can be overcome if staff and volunteers are alert to the need to consistently offer to take a patient to social areas and are prompt in responding to any patient's request for assistance in moving to where there are other people.

The least satisfactory arrangement probably is the semiprivate room. This gives neither the option for complete privacy nor the support of several other patients. When just two patients share a room, any personality conflicts are magnified and become important, rather than being diffused. In addition, when one roommate dies, it can be very stressful and frightening for the survivor. If there are several roommates, the death of one does not seem quite as overwhelming, nor does it have to be faced alone.

Of the existing inpatient facilities in the United States, several different room arrangements have been tried. Connecticut Hospice plans to use the English four-bed ward model plus private rooms. Hillhaven Hospice has semiprivate rooms which are used as private rooms when the census permits. Calvary Hospital in New York City opened its new building in 1978 with all private rooms—a change from the old building which had private rooms and wards of several sizes.

Until more experience with different room arrangements is gained in America, it seems safe to caution that the principal of maximum choice for the patient would argue for a choice of room arrangements (which can be administratively difficult) or for all private rooms. If experience in other settings can be generalized to the hospice setting, private rooms allow patients the most freedom and the most choice. Care must be taken with hospice patients who are not mobile to provide enough assistance so that patients can always act on a desire to leave their rooms and join other people in a social area.

The toilet and bathing areas should be built to the highest standards of accessibility and be easily negotiable by the patient, even when in a wheelchair. Adequate space should be available for staff or family members to provide assistance to the patient.

Lighting for patient rooms should be variable to permit accommodation to different uses and preferences. Direct ceiling lights, or lights so placed as to be uncomfortable for people in bed, should be avoided. Indirect or diffused lighting that can be augmented for reading or periods of visiting should be available.

All materials should be easily cleanable and durable, yet attention must be paid to choosing pleasing colors and textures and avoiding a sterile, institutional feeling. The designer may despair of these seemingly contradictory injunctions, yet materials meeting all these goals are available. For example, it is possible to find large easy chairs upholstered in washable vinyl with the look and texture of linen, an excellent blending of practicality and esthetics.

Every hospice room should have space for wheelchair storage so that the wheelchair can be easily reached but not provide an obstacle to family or staff.

Hospice buildings must meet all the codes for safety, but the safety features often symbolize the institutional environment. While exit signs, wide corridors, fire doors, and grab bars need to be included for patient safety, their institutional appearance can be offset by many homelike characteristics such as large plants, varied wall hangings, upholstered chairs, and carefully selected pieces of furniture in seating or conversational areas.

In a hospice, there is no need for extensive medical machinery. Hook-ups for sophisticated monitors and life-support systems are not necessary or appropriate. However, some patients will need oxygen in order to be comfortable, or suctioning, or an occasional intravenous feeding. Space for this equipment must be available at the bedside, but in a hospice program other items of comfort are equally, if not more, important. Adequate and abundant pillows should be within reach. Small tables on which to place a glass of juice and a pitcher of ice must be within reach of the patient. A place to put a book, a CB radio, a TV, or a pair of glasses must be near the bed. Storage for the patient's clothes and toiletries must be provided and accessible. In short, all the comforts that might be wished for in the sickroom must be planned and provided in an easily reachable place. Because so many of the individual's personal possessions will be small items, ample tabletop space should be provided adjacent to the bed. This could be on oversized over-bed tables, in shelves within easy reach, or on specially designed countertops adjacent to the bed.

Every opportunity should be provided to permit the patient to personalize the room with his own pictures and other prized possessions. It is unlikely that the patient will want to move large pieces of furniture other than perhaps a favorite chair. The dilemma presented for the institution is whether or not to furnish the area completely or to leave vacant walls and shelves for the patient. Perhaps a "library of furnishings" could be maintained from which the new patient could make selections as an alternative to bringing his own furnishings. Pictures, wall hangings, and bedspreads could be some of the items stocked. The patient should understand that personal belongings can be brought to the facility and that there is opportunity to choose some furnishings. The basic room design should support this policy.

One of the most important activities of hospice patients is receiving visitors. The patient's room must have adequate space for several, even many, visitors at a time. Comfortable places for everyone to sit should be provided. Space near the patient's bed as well as space a bit farther away should be available. This means that the rooms must be larger than the standard minimum for an inpatient facility, which allows an uncomfortable three-foot clearance around the bed—barely enough space for one chair to be pulled up to the head of the bed, let alone three, four, or five chairs. Especially in communities where ethnic groups tend toward large families, ten, fifteen, or more visitors may come at any one time. Unless having so many visitors is tiring and taxing to the patient, they should be encouraged, and there is no reason for the room design to inhibit them.

Providing a small patio outside each bedroom, either in a common patio area or as private patios, adds much to the comfort of the bedroom. The patio door, because of its ceiling to floor characteristic, permits a better visual span of the out-of-doors from bed or chair. If the patio has plantings, fountains, or bird feeders, there will be a variety of interesting attractions to watch. Having a patio close to the bed space will increase opportunities to spend some part of the day outside if the weather permits.

### ACOUSTICS

It is important that consideration be given to all the sources of distracting and disturbing sounds in the institutional environment. This is not to suggest that a noiseless environment is desirable, but rather to recommend elimination or control of harsh institutional sounds. For example, the hospice building should not have a paging system sounding messages throughout the building. Carts used to transport linen, food, medications, or cleaning equipment should have large rubber wheels that are clean and properly lubricated. A major noise producer is the fan-operated, individual room air-conditioning unit, which produces noises that interfere with normal social conversations. A careful study should be made of floor and wall treatments, acoustical surfaces, and sources of noise so that interior design can reduce the negative quality of institutional living.

### SPACE FOR FAMILIES

It almost goes without saying that there must be sufficient space and seating for family members in the patient's room. It is also desirable to be able to accommodate one or two people overnight in the patient's room or in a separate guest room. In one hospice two lounges furnished much like living rooms have couches that convert into beds. Each lounge has a bathroom so it easily becomes a self-contained guest room for a night or two. Linen is provided by the hospice, and family members feel free to make up the bed when it is needed. At the same hospice, family members sometimes stay overnight in the patient's bedroom. Low occupancy rates mean that often only one patient occupies a room meant for two. If the other bed is unoccupied, family members are welcome to use it, day or night. The fact that family members may choose to sleep in the patient's room or in a separate room, but still nearby, is optimal. At times a relative may not want to leave the room for even a minute. Others may need to get away in order to rest, yet do not want to be too far away. Down the hall is far enough away to be able to sleep untroubled by the patient's labored breathing, yet close enough to be called in the night if necessary.

The desires of family members to share physical intimacy should be respected and encouraged. This is another argument for private rooms. A private room furnished with a double bed makes it possible for a patient simply to close the door and request the staff to make no intrusion for some period of time.

Some rooms may be designed in the manner of an apartment or hotel suite with two adjacent, connecting rooms and individual toilet areas. The family portion of the suite could be furnished as a living room with couches convertible to beds. This room could be used by the family unit for visiting in a homelike, nonclinical environment as well as serve as the family sleeping space. The partition separating the two rooms should be easily movable to provide a large double room, space for large families, or easy access to the bed.

A small kitchen space would be useful for snacks, coffee, or heating a special dish brought from outside hospice. However, every effort should be made to avoid isolating the family in the privacy of their suite, unless this degree of privacy is desired. Opportunities for interacting with others in hospice should be provided.

Family members definitely need spaces within the hospice, other than the patient's bedroom, where they feel welcome. One hospice successfully converted two rooms originally planned to be patient rooms into lounges with a warm, living-room feeling. Both lounges are heavily used by staff, family visitors, and patients. The success of the lounges can be attributed to their location: each is near the middle of a patient corridor rather than isolated at the end of the corridor. Each comfortably seats six to eight people, large enough for a whole family but small enough to retain an intimate feeling. The decor of each—a throw rug, table lamps, couch, overstuffed chairs, plants, and pictures—gives a comfortable feeling. Diversions are also provided: one lounge has a TV, an aquarium, and a view onto the main-entrance courtyard with fountain; and the other has a small library, daily newspapers, board games, and a view onto a main street. These provide natural conversation starters for families, patients, and staff. Family members meet other family members, and staff members can interact naturally with patients and family.

Several small lounges are superior to one large lounge. Large lounges, unless broken up into smaller units by the furniture arrangement, tend to become a no man's land. The multipurpose room doesn't serve any purpose well. A small lounge suited to conversation will be used for that. Several small lounges also will allow several activities to go on at once. Children can watch TV while the doctor, adult relatives, and the chaplain confer in another room.

### KITCHEN

Often the heart of a family home, the kitchen is the gathering place as well as the source of aromas of food cooking and sights that increase anticipation of forthcoming food. Food is often an expression of love, the accompaniment of family celebrations and a ritual of regular family sharing. The hospice kitchen (provided for use by family and patients) should permit family meals and private dining. A stove and refrigerator should be available for cooking or reheating food prepared at home and brought to hospice. The aromas of a home-baked cake or pizza signal a family occasion in hospice or any home.

The kitchen area also can be a place to celebrate birthdays, have parties, or celebrate other occasions. Like other parts of the hospice facility, it should be accessible to persons in beds or wheelchairs and can be made especially inviting if it overlooks and is adjacent to an outdoor patio area.

### RELIGIOUS ACTIVITIES

Hospice care, because it offers a response to multiple personal needs, also must provide a religious program for its participants. Such a religious program should not be confined to the building; it can be offered at home through the outreach of the specialized staff.

Within the institutional building there should be a chapel as a focal point for individual or group worship. The chapel should be designed to be acceptable to most religious orientations as well as to those who want a peaceful place for reflection and worship without commitment to any specific religion. It should, of course, be accessible to people in wheelchairs or beds and accommodate family groups. It seems appropriate that the offices of the religious functionaries or chaplain be located in proximity to the chapel.

### VIEWING ROOM

A viewing room where family and friends can spend private time with the deceased prior to transfer to the mortuary should be provided. This is especially important where bedrooms are shared with other occupants. The viewing room should be decorated as a comfortable residential bedroom. Having the time, place, and privacy to say goodbye shortly after death seems especially important to family and is helpful in initiating the bereavement period. Location of the viewing room near the chapel and chaplain's office can help tie together religious expression at the time of death and be a source of comfort to the survivors. The viewing room provides the setting for an unhurried occasion to say goodbye at the time of death and to join together family and staff in this informal ritual. Such an opportunity to express deep personal feelings enables the bereaved to respond to the event of death and to prepare themselves for the activities to follow. It is an appreciated moment of quiet reflection and renewal. The viewing room should be located adjacent to the bedroom areas so that all may see the room and be aware of its availability and its intended use. By its presence it communicates a clear message of the spirituality of the hospice program and its pervasive regard for the individual and family.

## STAFF

It is consistent with the values of building a supportive community for staff that the building also provide a supportive environment in which staff can work. In addition to the concerns for comfortable working areas, adequacy of supplies, and proximity to patients, equipment, and supplies, the building should provide areas where staff can retreat and restore their capacities and resume their efforts.

Staff should not be discouraged, either by institutional policy or design, from integrating into patient and family activities where it is not intrusive into family privacy. Taking a break with a family, or joining in lunch with a patient, may be an expression of closeness that should not be discouraged. But staff should also have the option to withdraw to the privacy of a quiet room for reflection, or to a comfortable staff lounge to join with other staff away from patients and families. Comfortable furniture, access to coffee and other snacks, the availability of a pleasant outdoor patio should be part of the staff environment. Staff dealing with and experiencing the deaths of those they care for need comfortable spaces to relax, get away from the pressure, and under some circumstances just to let off steam from the trauma of loss. The staff dining area and education training areas should be similarly supportive of morale. The facility should communicate to staff members that they are important and should signal special appreciation for their needs in the hospice environment.

## CHILDREN

The presence of children, their sounds, their loving, their inquisitiveness and playfulness add much to any environment. Children should be encouraged to be at home at hospice. One way to achieve this would be to provide children's play areas with games and toys and outdoor recreational areas easily reached and shared by hospice residents.

Some hospice buildings provide child-care quarters and programs for children of employees, both to assist staff and to encourage the presence of children in the hospice environment.

## Summary

The hospice design should be small in scale and size to approximate closely a homelike environment. All necessary safety and convenience features must be provided for patients and staff, but these can be offset by a decor featuring warmth of colors, fabrics, and furnishings.

Special attention must be given to the individual's preference for privacy or for sharing of a bedroom. Families should always be welcome and the space, both for day and night use, should give evidence of their importance in the program.

Staff also must be given the option for privacy and distance from work during brief periods. Adequate staff retreat areas will enhance the staff's capacity to work comfortably in the hospice environment.

# 7

# Administration of a Hospice Program
## Funding and Licensure

*The Hospice concept is so innovative that the task of
creating and staffing a structure to deal effectively with the
needs of the terminally ill and their families was
formidable. Two fundamental difficulties faced—and
continue to confront—the New Haven Hospice: first, the
status quo for terminal care in the American medical
community, and second, the problem of fitting Hospice
into the bureaucratic maze of American health care
without changing its purposes and nature.*

*Despite the benefits of the Hospice program to
patients and families, these characteristics make Hospice
care a square peg to be fitted into the round holes of
Medicare, Medicaid, certification, various reimbursement
plans, and physician referral systems. In addition,
considerable misunderstanding and ignorance within
the community itself often creates a distorted picture
of Hospice.*

Sylvia A. Lack and Robert W. Buckingham III
in *First American Hospice*

DAVID ENGLISH (1978), in a presentation sponsored by the Catholic Hospital Association, described how he perceived hospital administrators would feel when faced with the problems of financing a hospice program. He used an analogy to the stages of grief and bereavement often cited in literature related to death and dying.

*Stage 1—Shock.* They won't believe the size of the deficit. Numbness will set in.

*Stage 2—Emotional release,* probably expressed in great anger towards you.

*Stage 3—Depression,* sadness, a feeling of being overwhelmed.

*Stage 4—Great physical symptoms,* especially loss of appetite.

*Stage 5—Anxiety.* Try to remind him that wrestling with this problem is not all bad. It can be helpful to his long term, productive life.

*Stage 6—Anger.* Anger at insurance companies, anger at the federal government, anger at you.

*Stage 7—Guilt* about the way he felt and the extent of his anger.

*Stage 8—Resistance.* Resist giving up. However, I am not sure whether it is necessarily appropriate to tell him to let God take over.

*Stage 9—Hope* gradually comes through.

*Stage 10—Reaffirm reality.*

It is encouraging to note that in this realistic process that which begins with shock can end with hope and reality. It is also good to be forewarned about potential problems new groups may have to face in developing a sound footing for a new hospice program.

## Administrative Flexibility: Responsiveness to Those Being Served

Management of hospice shares common objectives with all organizations. Essential to any successful operation are good management of personnel, funding and budgeting, and controls. In addition, hospice management must be responsive to the unique service character of the organization. Organizational goals must be reached, but the style and character of their achievement must reflect the service needs of hospice. It seems appropriate to generalize that hospice needs sound management but must be organized in an open system that is flexible and responsive to change, making it possible to achieve stated objectives by directing human and other resources to those ends.

Hospice must have a special involvement in the community because of its unique role and service. Hospice should not compete with nor challenge the roles of nursing homes, hospitals, or home health agencies, but rather develop relationships with these health agencies in order to interpret the unique service of hospice. When it becomes clear that other health agencies are unable to provide comparable care for the terminally ill, hospice care will be recognized for its unique quality. This has already happened in many communities where hospice care has been established.

**Principle:** *Hospice management must combine the management functions of any health care organization with flexibility and responsiveness to the needs of dying persons.*

**Discussion:** An orderly sequence of steps should be taken by a new hospice group to assure a successful hospice project. At the outset the early supporters of the program should identify the sponsors and determine the nature of the sponsoring authority. For example, there may be a hospice planning committee of interested persons who will incorporate as the board of directors of the hospice program. Alternatively, the planning committee may be a subgroup of an existing organization such as a hospital, church, or university or may be a staff committee of an existing health care organization exploring hospice care.

This beginning organization may include a professional staff person or may distribute tasks to its volunteer members for completion. At some point the group may want to involve resources from other hospice programs to assist in development of their own program or employ an appropriate consultant to provide direction and staff support.

An early assignment for the group members will be to acquaint themselves with the hospice literature and evolve their own philosophy of hospice care that is responsive to the sponsor group and is compatible with the national standards of the hospice movement. The group should be in touch with the National Hospice Organization as well as other hospice groups for an understanding of the philosophy and organizational structure of other hospice groups.

The group should then be ready to consider issues relating to program content. Will there be inpatient as well as home care? Will some services be provided by other organizations under contract, or will the hospice organization be directly responsible for its own services? At this point the full scope of hospice services should be understood and a plan designed both for the range of services to be offered and for the most appropriate entry point to initiate services. Unless a group is assured of an established commitment to inpatient care, perhaps through a hospital

wanting to utilize a portion of its physical plant for hospice care, it may
be wise to initiate its program through a small home-care service.

In this case a decision must be made whether to affiliate with an ongoing home-care program or to initiate an entirely new program. An all
new program will have to provide for paid staff and determine procedures
for payment for services. An application will have to be made to license
the program. This begins with the application of a certificate of need made
to the local health systems agency (described in this chapter) and will
require a responsible corporate structure in the state.

The group may, however, exercise another option and provide volunteer services to demonstrate the value of hospice care. In either case—a
corporate structure or volunteer services—the group offering hospice care
should be thoroughly trained in the elements of hospice care so that only
highly competent professional services will be provided. To assist in assuring compliance with organizational philosophy and hospice standards,
policy statements should be prepared for the services to be provided; for
the personnel to be engaged, whether volunteers or paid; and for the
collateral relationships with any related service agency likely to interface
with hospice.

The group should then establish criteria for admission into the program
and the application and assessment procedure to be used to obtain the
hospice services.

Following these steps and adhering to the hospice principles identified
in this document will enable the group to make the transition from a
conceptual idea to a practical program. As with all practical programs,
the sponsor will have to deal with the issues of funding and licensing an
ongoing program.

### Management Plan

A sound management plan appropriate to a hospice program will require
that people and money be managed in accordance with necessary rules
and regulations, and still encourage community involvement. Management of buildings may or may not be part of the administrator's responsibilities, depending upon the organizational location of the hospice program. Under all circumstances, appropriate funding will be essential to
implement the hospice program.

At present the rules of licensing and funding hospice programs are
not supportive of a comprehensive hospice program. Home care is
governed by license requirements, rules, and reimbursement procedures
that are different from those for inpatient services; and only very limited
resources support day care/night care or bereavement services. Hospice
programs must expect financial struggles until society changes licensing

regulations to recognize and support the new services of a comprehensive hospice program.

The clear implication is that a new hospice program should seek financial support from sources other than the traditional health care reimbursements since the traditional third-party payment resources must be augmented. Funding new hospice programs will be difficult. Hospice programs being developed need to understand the critical issues of funding and licensing and seek to alleviate these problems by working for the acceptance of hospice care by additional state legislatures, state health departments, Blue Cross plans, and other insurance companies.

John Hackley, president of the Hillhaven Foundation, sponsor of Hillhaven Hospice, and board member of the National Hospice Organization, recently wrote for *Hospital Progress* a discussion of the issues of funding and licensure. With his permission and that of *Hospital Progress,* his important article is included here in its entirety.

## Financing and Accrediting Hospices *

A review of the evolution of the U.S. health-care delivery system clearly confirms that general availability of a specific service tends to follow the existence of third-party reimbursement for that service. This realization, at first blush, implies that hospice care is fundamentally dependent on monetary considerations.

Conversely, the planning, design, and implementation of a single hospice program may not depend primarily on fiscal considerations, given the unique conditions of that single program. But if the hospice concept of care is critically important and therefore should be broadly available in the U.S. health-care delivery system, financial feasibility becomes a fundamental concern.

### EFFECTS OF THE BRITISH HOSPICE MODEL

The United States has benefited substantially from the British experience in the development, proliferation, and perfection of hospice care for terminally ill persons and their families. Documented British experience has contributed significantly to the development of U.S. hospice programs in such critical areas as medical direction, pain control, symptom control, palliative care, medical protocols, psychosocial needs, spiritual support, and bereavement services for patients and families. Similarly, the British experience has facilitated understanding of the sensitivity required in recruitment, orientation, continuing education, and emotional support for hospice personnel, both staff and volunteer.

Perhaps the difficulty in translating the British hospice model to the U.S. milieu can be attributed to the reluctance or inability of some U.S. hospice advocates to appreciate the very real differences between the medical-economic characteristics of the two countries' health-care delivery systems. Hospice care in Great Britain is available regardless of the terminally ill patient's ability to pay for the care. Great Britain, however, has a National Health Service that reimburses the hospice program. Obviously, in the United States there is no such nationwide health service and therefore no preexisting assurance of reimbursement for hospice care.

One could assume that in the United States there is no attitudinal objection to providing hospice care as an option to any person who qualifies for the program and chooses it. It is imperative that the society recognize and accept hospice care and enact the necessary legislation to ensure governmental and private coverage of hospice care. Hospice programs will then be assured of necessary, reasonable reimbursement for care regardless of the personal resources of the terminally ill patient and the family.

An analysis of the history of third-party coverage for other generally recognized modalities of care reveals this series of steps:

Professional acceptance of a new modality
   leads to
Development of a universally accepted definition of the service and the
Development of criteria and standards of performance, quality, and
   eligibility
   leads to
Programs of licensure, certification, and accreditation
   leads to
Significant public demand for the service
   leads to
Government agencies' extension of partial or full coverage of the
   service (Medicare or Medicaid)
   leads to
Private and other third-party extension of partial or full coverage of
   the service
   leads to
Substantially universal coverage of the service
   leads to
Proliferation of the service until it is considered "generally available"

The current interest in humanization of care reduces the likelihood of prolonged resistance to payment for the hospice care option. The society may—through equitable financing, reimbursement, and other fiscal incentives—promote the availability of this care option to a substantial number of citizens.

Ideally, four facets of care are found in a comprehensive hospice service: Home care predominates, and inpatient twenty-four-hour-a-day care serves as a back-up. The day-and-night care option allows the program to be adaptable to the patient's immediate needs. And bereavement service is available for surviving family members.

SIX CRITICAL PROBLEMS

Consideration of the financial feasibility and viability of hospice services should address six critical problems. A reimbursement policy for comprehensive hospice care should cover the following:

First, licensure obviously will significantly affect reimbursement and the financial feasibility of any developing hospice program within the foreseeable future. The nature of the individual hospice program's license is related primarily to what will develop as the inpatient twenty-four-hour-a-day service component. Existing hospice models range from the hospital-based service to one beginning with a good hospice home-care service or even one developed within the framework of volunteer organizations that provide a "friendly visitor" type of service. A few facilities, each with slightly different features, are developing a "special hospital-hospice" state licensure category. I prefer this approach even though it is obviously a complex, tedious process. Otherwise, the hospice program may be distorted into one of the traditional licensure models by using licensure standards and criteria that were developed for established institutional categories such as skilled nursing care or the acute hospital.

Second, under existing reimbursement programs death is not an allowable treatment objective. And rehabilitation is still interpreted at the federal level in the traditional vocational rehabilitation model. Therefore, rehabilitation, understood as prevention of deformities or deterioration or as maintenance of a patient's present level of function, is not a valid objective.

Third, a multilevel care program that permits patients to alternate among levels of care according to need creates constant exceptions to standard, regimented "covered" programs of care. Any such program creates enormous problems for traditional reimbursement programs with their customary eligibility criteria, admission and discharge processes, standard records, and "level of care" determination processes.

Fourth, some hospice advocates seem inclined to approach reimbursement at this early stage like a militant group with the "only social conscience." Such persons perceive third parties as unenlightened because "they" won't voluntarily rush to pour money into hospice care—care which has not been adequately defined, for which universally agreed upon standards and criteria have not been formulated, and for which there still is no body of accumulated actuarial experience in this country upon which to predicate any reasonable payment mechanism or insurable coverage plan. Third parties, whether public or private, are just as obligated to be conscientious custodians of the funds entrusted to them for the purchase of care as are hospice service providers obligated to the recipients of care.

Fifth, evidence has not been evaluated nor is there research into the necessary hospice care roles and the benefits of heretofore unallowable costs such as those for nonclinical services considered essential in a comprehensive hospice program. In addition, the concept of the patient together with family as the unit of care has far-reaching implications for state and federal reimbursement programs as well as for other third-party coverage. For example, is bereavement coverage a matter of allowing reimbursement for a service cost incurred after the death of the insured? Raising this question may seem like insensitivity to some, but for those in public agencies and for private third parties these are real considerations of conscience. The resolution of the question of bereavement coverage has greater implications for third parties than did the precedent they set in reimbursing aspects of hospice care during the early days of the movement.

Sixth, arbitrarily defining skilled care affects reimbursement policies. At issue is the provision under the Medicare program particularly and also under state-administered Medicaid programs that the covered person must require skilled care. The Social Security Administration has gradually given a more and more restrictive interpretation of the federal definition of skilled care. Essentially this interpretation has moved toward precise, measurable clinical tasks associated with cure and has totally disregarded the nature of care required in serving the total person. Ironically, the Medicare standards for certification repeatedly call for the interdisciplinary approach to patient care, presumably to ensure the evolution of dynamic, constructive, and effective care.

SETTING STANDARDS AND MONITORING

None of these obstructions to early and broadly applicable reimbursement of hospice service appears insurmountable. The public's awareness of hospice care is accelerating at such an unprecedented rate that public impatience with the customary lag in changing policy may be anticipated.

Satisfying public interest in the early acceptance of hospice care as a universally recognized option for terminally ill persons and concurrently providing broadly available reimbursement for hospice care require that at least four critical developments be addressed immediately: 1) a precise, generally accepted definition of hospice and of the constellation of professional services that represent the irreducible minimum constituting hospice care; 2) a nationally accepted guide to licensure standards that could be used as a model for individual states to follow in formalizing licensure rules, regulations, and expectations and in formulating monitoring mechanisms; 3) a set of accreditation standards or some other evaluative tool that could be objectively applied and that government and other third parties could rely on for assurance that a program bearing the name "hospice" does, in fact, provide a discernibly unique hospice service; 4) particularly for the Medicare-Medicaid programs, the development of eligibility requirements that an individual must meet in order to qualify for hospice care coverage by Medicare-Medicaid. The fourth item is particularly critical in covering hospice care for older people, since other private third parties may initially hold back to follow the Medicare lead. Medicare-Medicaid could provide an actuarial cushion for coverage of the high-risk older people who need hospice care, and thus other third parties would find extension of coverage actuarially feasible.

If these four sets of standard setting and monitoring tools are to be developed in a thoughtful, sophisticated, sound, and effective way, their formulation will benefit from input from more than the federal reimbursement agencies and the relatively few existing hospice services. Established national provider organizations have a real obligation to join in the action at this critical, formative time in U.S. hospice history.

## VALUABLE SUPPORT FROM NATIONAL ASSOCIATIONS

The National Hospice Organization (NHO) has provided unprecedented leadership to this exploding national movement. As an organization of hospice programs, hospice advocates, and hospice experts in the United States, it has potential for the sound direction of this rapidly expanding resource for terminally ill persons and their families. If hospice care is to be integrated appropriately into the fabric of the nation's health-care delivery system, organizations of the various medical and health care professionals and providers must collaborate to assure that hospice care in this country does not fall victim to American faddism.

Acceptance and properly directed support of hospice care as an essential component of the national health-care delivery system by the national associations of health care professions and provider organizations could do much to protect the integrity and uniqueness of the hospice concept. Additionally, the cooperation and wisdom of these same national organizations underpinning the dynamic NHO leadership increase the prospect of early recognition of hospice care as a reimbursable modality option. Unless hospice care is reimbursable, the number of professionally sound hospice service programs adequate for meeting even presently known need may fail to develop.

## THE IMPOSSIBILITY OF FREE CARE

A financial management consultant, speaking recently at the Third National Hospice Conference at Dominican College, San Rafael, California, startled his audience with the comment that "now, the trouble with hospice people is that they think nonprofit." This observation is consistent with the comments of other experts, who know that there is no such thing as a free service. Any health care must have a source of support.

There is possibly one unfortunate consequence of the fact that a few early hospice programs have had total outside support. That circumstance was great for them; and the funding organizations were highly motivated, and rightfully so, in trying to encourage the development of a highly desirable model of care. This history of early support may leave many people with the impression that hospice care should be free. But we are not going to have hospice care in the United States if we approach hospice development with that attitude, because it is not feasible. Certainly hospice care should be available to those who cannot pay for it, but it does have to be supported by some constant, reliable source. Subsequent programs will always benefit from the experience of the few original programs that were fortunate enough in their sponsorship to begin by providing free care; but the majority of programs—those that endure—will be ones that were fiscally sound in conception and operation.

Historically in the United States services have tended to follow the availability of health care dollars. Because of the unprecedented public interest and growing demand for hospice care, hospices may well be the first major exception to that pattern. Early hospice programs are the work of a nucleus of pioneers to whom fell an obligation to develop services and document experience. Upon that foundation, or data base, the society can soundly predicate an equitable approach to regulating and financing this most humane segment of the national health-care delivery system.

• • •

Hackley identifies the importance of licensure as the first of six critical issues and says, "Licensure will significantly affect reimbursement and the financial feasibility of any developing hospice program" (1979).

There are several approaches to licensing hospice programs. These include:

1. The hospice home-care program will probably be licensed as a home-care agency or the services will be provided by agreement with a licensed home-care agency. This would make possible provision of the basic hospice service, but would not provide for an integration of home care into other related hospice services under a common license or funding mechanism.

   This approach might also encounter difficulties in justifying care of the dying person or bereavement services as part of the reimbursable home-care services.

2. The hospice inpatient program could be organized within a licensed hospital or nursing home and be covered by the host organizations' institutional license. However, the continuum of noninstitutional services as well as payment for the quality and quantity of services

for dying persons might be challenged by the third-party payer as inappropriate to the institutional license.

3. A hospital institutional program could be licensed as a distinct hospital, meeting all the regulations required of a hospital and receiving reimbursement for hospital care. This generally would not cover the noninstitutional characteristics of the program, and its feasibility would depend upon the hospital's having the flexibility to relax traditional hospital regulations not appropriate to care of the terminally ill.

4. The hospice program could also be licensed as a special hospital, a licensing category available in some states. This has been used to license hospitals limiting admission to patients requiring care or treatment for substance abuse, rehabilitative medicine, psychiatric treatment, or other special services that do not need to conform to all the regulations of a general hospital. This approach would be preferable to licensing hospice as a skilled nursing care facility, a most inappropriate category, but would not permit including home care and bereavement services as part of a coordinated program.

5. The most desirable approach to hospice licensing would be a special category supportive of the comprehensive definition of hospice and permitting inclusion of outpatient services, home care, and bereavement counseling as parts of the single, comprehensive license for hospice care.

If they are to provide appropriate reimbursement for hospice care, the state and federal governments will need to accept hospice as a discrete level of care in the health care continuum, with reimbursement rates established for hospice based on the content of hospice services. Hospice will have to connote a consistent program content throughout the country so that standards can be applied and services appropriately licensed and reimbursed.

## Health Systems Agency

Another important aspect of community involvement requires that hospice develop an understanding relationship with the health systems agency of the local community. Health care administrators are probably very much aware of the problems and requirements of meeting the health systems agency expectations. Hospice administrators may not yet, but, because hospice programs are essentially health care programs, they must also conform to the same health planning expectations.

Every health care service must apply to the health systems agency for a "certificate of need," an authorization to offer the service and approval for the state to license the service. If hospice care is to be considered by the health systems agency, the community health plan must not only specify hospice service but must also quantify units of care and scope of service. The initial step, then, is to see that hospice is introduced into the local health plan and to interpret the program so that the health plan will support the full scope of hospice programs. The hospice program will have to be written into the local plan in a way that is compatible with the state licensing regulations. Hospice promoters have to take a dual approach of promoting, both at the local health systems agency level and at the state health department level.

Because hospice is relatively new in our society and because few data exist supporting the experiences of a full hospice program, it is difficult to interpret the program to policy makers. While many policy makers have read about hospice programs, few have had actual experience with the service, and most have only a beginning awareness of hospice potential from the media or health care journal articles. It would be appropriate for the emerging hospice program to prepare a portfolio of current information about hospice, including standards and definitions provided by the National Hospice Organization. Personal conversations and presentations to policy makers are also helpful, and where possible a tour of an existing hospice program should be arranged. It also could be very valuable to develop a community conference or workshop about hospice, sponsored by the local hospice group. Every effort should be made to arrange the workshop so that local policy makers can participate. Guest speakers or workshop leaders could be personnel from existing hospice programs. The event could attract media attention around the presence of a noted guest speaker. Private meetings for policy makers could also be held, with hospice workshop staff to interpret the program, describe personal experiences, and answer the questions that would be sure to arise. A listing of hospice programs is available from the National Hospice Organization.

The planning process described above is one that most new hospice programs have successfully utilized. When the first hospice programs were developing in this country, they were reliant on hospice people from England to provide the models and initiatives. While Dr. Cicely Saunders and other colleagues from England are most capable of inspiring new hospice programs in this country, there are now sufficient programs in various parts of this country to make it possible to find an experienced American to talk about hospice.

After hospice has been incorporated into the local health systems agency plan and recognized in the rules and regulations of the state health department, the local hospice can apply for a certificate of need and will rely for guidance in this process on the local health systems agency. There undoubtedly will be forms to complete and public hearings to attend, at which time the goals and scope of the program can be defended. However, prior to the public hearing, the hospice concept should be interpreted to policy makers or the hearing group by the hospice planning group. In this way the hospice application can be reviewed with knowledge and appreciation for the content of the program, its staffing, and funding requirements.

A new hospice will also have to appear before the health systems agency in order to establish the charges for services. Any subsequent change in charges or significant change in the scope of the program must similarly be defended before the agency. It should be apparent that hospice management will need to spend considerable time with the local health systems agency. Because the policy makers in the health systems agency generally are actively involved in community affairs, the ongoing interpretation of hospice to the community is an especially important management function that should be appropriately provided for in the assignments of hospice staff and volunteers.

## Funding

Every hospice should be developed with a funding plan to utilize to the fullest the existing resources and to identify funding gaps that must be overcome either in the planning for services or in the advocacy for new resources. The newness of hospice and its limited payment experiences strongly suggest that the status quo not be accepted as the ultimate funding arrangement. Success in obtaining new funding will to a large extent depend upon the community relations established by hospice and the ability to interpret the importance of the program, offering comparisons with existing services and costs. As such, the initial community involvement plan also becomes the program to identify financial resources and to interpret the need for funding hospice care.

The funding strategy should examine the following sources (English, 1978):

- Reimbursement and fee for service.
- Shared services.
- Federal government.
- State government.
- County/city government.
- Foundations.
- Corporations/associations.
- Employee or union funds.
- Other organizations, i.e., churches.
- Private individuals.
- General public.

It will be useful to recognize the difference between funding requirements for start-up and ongoing funding. Examination should also be made of those services that can be expected to be funded through ongoing resources versus those ongoing services for which there is no immediate source of funding.

It should be helpful to group current funding resources into the following categories to better understand the parts of the funding requirement to which they can respond:

1. *Philanthropic support.* This often serves as the base for seed money, start-up funds, and special projects. However, local community gifts, church support, or family foundations may provide the ongoing money to meet the nonreimbursed service costs.
2. *Governmental support.* Funds may be available from federal, state, or local governments for construction, for initial start-up, or for special projects to serve a designated underserved population of the community. Federal agencies that have funded hospice programs or hospice-related activities are The National Cancer Institute, The Administration on Aging, The National Institute on Aging, Health Care Finance Administration, and The National Institute of Mental Health.
3. *Reimbursement for service.* The major reimbursement resources are the Medicare and Medicaid programs. At this time these two programs should provide the mainstay of ongoing funding. It is also possible to combine the Medicaid (Title 19) program, which pays for health services, with Title 20, whose scope is limited to the social services. Title 20 may be the source of payments for family counseling, bereavement, and homemaker services, while Title 19 covers the approved health care portion of physician services, pharmaceuticals, home health care, and institutional care (Gibson, 1978).

What appears to be required is "creative funding," or the utilization of a broad range of resources put together in a management program for hospice. Important also is the need to interpret hospice to prospective providers in order to add to the existing resources.

Advocacy for new funds will be strengthened by the availability of data to support the viability of hospice care. Gibson (1978) recommends that the following data should be compiled and used to garner support:

1. Historical costs.
2. Patient origin studies.
3. Projected caseload and costs.
4. Existing or planned relationship with other providers.
5. Related experiences of other hospice programs.

## Management Committees

Earlier, in the chapter dealing with staff, four levels of staff meetings were described. These included:

1. In-service education.
2. Case management for home care and inpatient services.
3. Administrative staff meetings.
4. Community support meetings.

Additionally, management will be involved in a number of management committees designed to permit a high level of staff participation in management functions. One of the major assignments of management staff will be to provide leadership for the governing board or community advisory board, depending upon the organizational design.

1. The *Governing Board* establishes policies for the organization, provides a liaison with the community, interprets policies to the community, and may be involved in fund raising. Where this is an advisory board to some other governing body, there may be recommendations for policy adoption rather than responsibility to adopt policies. This board may meet monthly or quarterly, depending upon whether it is a policy or an advisory group.
2. The *Executive Committee* is composed of department heads or senior staff members of the hospice who meet with the administration weekly to review the overall conduct of the hospice program. This group should concern itself with management problems, staff turnover, interdepartmental activities, and long-range planning.
3. The *Employee Council,* composed of representatives of all levels of hospice staff, should meet monthly to review personnel practices and policies and to make recommendations for change to the administrator.
4. The *Bereavement Committee* should meet weekly to review the bereavement caseload, identify bereavement problems, and to make staff assignments for bereavement services.
5. The *Committee on Privacy and Confidentiality* should meet as needed to review all requests for research, special students, or assignment of practicum students.
6. The *Community Education Committee* should meet weekly to schedule community speaking engagements, coordinate tours and visits to the program, and evaluate the community contacts and services. This committee should be responsible for preparing brochures, newsletters, and news releases.
7. The *Safety Committee* should meet monthly to survey the inpatient facility for potential hazards, to review the accident record, and to

make recommendations for in-service education to correct any deficiencies.

8. The *Infection Control Committee* should meet quarterly to review any problems with infectious diseases and to authorize studies of the environment to reduce any infection hazards.

9. The *Pharmacy Committee* should meet quarterly with the consultant pharmacist to review the drug use, administration of drugs, and drug problems.

While this listing of management committees may not exhaust the possibilities, it is intended to suggest the variety of responsibilities for hospice programs that should be shared with the entire staff through an organized committee structure.

## Community

Hospice must anticipate a long process of building community interests and supports that will ultimately lead to its acceptance in the health care network. Specific staff and volunteer time should be assigned to build a strong base of interest and commitment in the community. This will ultimately lead to appropriate licensing and funding and with that, the ability to provide hospice care on an ongoing basis.

**Principle:** *The newness of hospice in most communities and its dependence upon broad-based community support require that new hospice programs be developed with a strong community orientation.*

**Discussion:** Hospice is dependent upon health professionals, primarily physicians, for referrals and must gain the support of these health professionals. Because hospice is a new concept, there is considerable uncertainty about its role and its competition with other established health services for clientele, money, staff, and community support. The newness and attractiveness of the hospice idea will evoke careful examination, if not cautious skepticism, from the traditional health providers. Hospice care must ultimately be viewed as an extension of existing health care and as a complement to the current scheme of acute and long-term care systems. As such, each of the levels of health care (acute, long-term, and hospice) will complement the others and contribute to a more sophisticated and appropriate health-care delivery system. Because hospice will not stand alone, but will be part of a total community health program, it must be initiated with appropriate community understanding and supports.

Hospice also represents an advance in the community's readiness to deal with issues of death and dying. As a program of caring, hospice is a visible expression of the concern and discussion about care of the dying.

Hospice, then, represents a community's readiness to act in a specific way and thus becomes a symbol of the community's caring for the dying. Because of hospice's relationship to the community and the values it represents, the community, through its educational institutions, churches, service groups, and others will want to observe hospice, see what it does, and better understand its role. Many in the community will seek an affiliation with hospice because of their own personal experiences with loss; others will find in hospice a new opportunity for service or religious expression. Community interest in hospice will be high, and hospice will need to provide opportunities for visits, study, and affiliation.

The hospice program should be viewed as having the responsibility of improving care of the dying throughout the community. To achieve this goal, an active educational program for health care providers can be offered by hospice. In a sense, the hospice is the laboratory demonstrating how care of the dying can be improved. Classes can be offered for a single discipline or can represent an interdisciplinary mix, and should be offered to physicians, nurses, social workers, and chaplains throughout the community.

## Protection of Privacy

Many groups and individuals will want to visit the hospice building to see firsthand the environment provided for the dying. As a result, hospice staff will be asked to serve both the hospice occupant and the student. There should be no equivocation of the primary responsibility to the dying person. Arrangements will have to be made to accommodate visitors at the convenience of staff and residents of hospice. Needs of the residents must be the primary concern; staff time, which ultimately means budget, should be allocated to education only after there is certainty that the needs of the dying persons are being met appropriately.

Management has special responsibility to protect the privacy and confidentiality of the persons using hospice. While this is so for all health care programs, it becomes more critical for hospice because of the need to demonstrate the importance of this service. Hospices, their programs, staff and service groups will be examined and studied very intensively, as community interest increases. Seeking to know the values and potentials of hospice programs, both local and out-of-town visitors will seek out existing hospices for new ideas and new models after which to pattern their programs. The institutionalized hospice occupant is in no position either to restrict hospice visitors or to withdraw from the hospice building. Because of their dependency, some patients may respond positively to management's requests for permission to allow outsiders to visit or study the hospice program. Some may be too weak and frail to become involved.

Privacy and confidentiality must be a primary responsibility of staff. There may be requests to conduct studies or research, and there will undoubtedly be ongoing conflict between the need of concerned persons to learn more about hospice to improve care of the dying and the rights of privacy and confidentiality of the patients. Reich (1978) offers "three ethical principles commonly applied to the moral dilemmas in human research." These include:

1. The principle of beneficence requires that the research effort should ultimately produce good and prevent harm,
2. The principle of just distribution or in the comparative treatment of individuals, requires a fair and equitable distribution of benefits and burdens, and finally,
3. The principle of respect for persons requires that the dignity and autonomy of persons be promoted and protected.

In order to insure protection of the dignity and autonomy of the individual, all studies, research interviews, and taking of photographs should be preceded by informed consent and be entirely voluntary. The individual should have a complete written and verbal explanation of the project, have assurance that his refusal to participate in the project will not in any way endanger his care within hospice, and should be permitted to withdraw from the agreement at any time.

A designated period for community visitors should be scheduled at a time when the program can be introduced and described through interactions between visitors and staff. Use of appropriate audiovisual techniques permits showing the entire facility without intruding on the privacy of the occupants. Dying persons don't come to hospice to be put on display. They choose hospice for care. Hospice responsibilities for education cannot be justified if they entail intrusion into the privacy of the dying person.

Responsibilities for arranging the educational tours and classes and interpretation of the program can be assigned to a specially trained group of volunteers to reduce direct staff involvement.

Some students interested in hospice may seek an internship, residence, or special field assignment involving an intensive schedule of activities, providing service to the program as they complete an educational experience. These students should have a tutorial or preceptor relationship with a member of the hospice professional staff, i.e., a counseling student working directly with the counseling staff. These students become the direct teaching responsibility of the professional staffperson and for the duration of their experience should be considered hospice staff, conforming to all expectations of staff performance appropriate to any staff person in a comparable position.

## Committee on Privacy and Confidentiality

The more successful the hospice program proves to be in providing care, developing stature and positive reputation, and achieving community support, the more it will be subject to potential intrusion on the privacy of its occupants through visits, new interests, television interviews, and reports of a variety of journals and magazines. Hospice will have to find a creative way of enhancing its image without compromising its responsibilities to its service group. One way this can be anticipated and handled would be to establish a hospice committee on privacy and confidentiality, or what might also be known as an institutional review board. This group should be composed of hospice staff and members of the community and should have a physician, chaplain, social worker, and nurse as the basic membership. Every effort should be made to include the services of family members who have used the hospice program or who are current users of the program.

The committee should prepare a statement of expectations regarding privacy and confidentiality and identify how community requests for visits, research, or other studies will be reviewed. Guidelines for acceptable requests should be available to all who make the request to use the hospice program as a learning opportunity.

The community should not be discouraged from using hospice and benefiting from the program. Advances in caring for dying patients should be shared so that all who live may be comforted by knowing how some may die. Constraints should be established to protect the patients, but the community should be welcomed into hospice.

## Summary

Hospice administration must be concerned with developing and offering a new level of health service for which very few models currently exist. This requires a greater degree of creativity than might be expected from an administrator experienced in another level of health care.

One major area of responsibility will relate to the management of people, a subject discussed in an earlier chapter. Concern should be given to the way the organization is structured in order to carry out its stated objectives. The unique characteristics of hospice needing consideration here are: 1) the small size of hospice and the importance of accommodating organizational structure to small size, 2) the need to maintain close, even intimate, relationships with the persons using the service, 3) having flexibility in meeting the individual needs of each participant, and 4) sensitivity to the continuing stress of staff and volunteers as they regularly deal with death and loss and provide support to survivors.

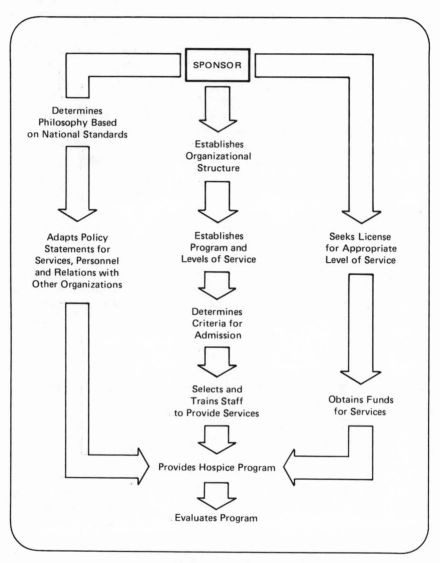

**Figure 7-1**   The Process for Developing a New Hospice Program

Additionally, it should be expected that major energies will have to be allocated to the areas of community relations, licensing, and funding. Obviously, without community support and financial resources hospice would not exist. While all organizations need community support and finances, because hospice has not yet been integrated into the health care system as a sharer of funding resources, it must chart its own course to assure support. There has obviously been a high community acceptance of the need for this new way of caring for dying persons. Such acceptance must now be backed up with financing that will permit fulfillment of the promise hospice offers.

The process described for developing a new hospice program is summarized in Figure 7–1.

# 8

## Evaluation of Hospice Programs
### Some Methodological Considerations

Robert William Buckingham

THERE EXISTS a most urgent need in the field of terminal care and hospice program development for applied evaluative research. This evaluative research must concern itself with utilizing biomedical and social science methodology.

Increasing demands for greater accountability are currently affecting the field of terminal care and hospice development. Substantiating evidence in support of any more expansion or development in hospice programs is lacking. Henceforth, we must concentrate our present and future efforts on building adequate and appropriate evaluation methodologies and practices for existing and developing hospice programs.

## What Is Program Evaluation?

To the extent that judgment is involved in decision making, evaluation is taking place. Administrators, planners, and providers are involved in evaluational activities on a daily basis. The decision to hire or fire an employee, to expand facilities, and to introduce a new product are all evaluative decisions. What distinguishes program evaluation from day-to-day evaluative decisions is the use of the *scientific method*. The essence of the scientific method is the attempt to isolate causes of particular events or outcomes. If a particular hospice program appears to be associated with a beneficial effect, one must know whether the effect can really be attributable to the program operation or whether it might result from some other external factor.

## Hospice Health-Policy Analysis

Hospice health-policy analysis should be the first priority of any developing hospice program. Hospice health-policy analysis involves the drawing

*Editor's note:* Dr. Robert Buckingham, co-author of *First American Hospice,* was recently appointed to the faculty of the Department of Policy, Planning and Administration and the Department of Family Medicine at the University of Arizona. He has served on the staff of the New Haven Hospice, New Haven, Connecticut, for three years, and as a consultant to other hospice programs. He was asked to prepare the final chapter of this book from the perspective of a medical researcher who recognizes the critical importance of objective evaluation of any human services program, particularly one newly emerging as a competitor for public support.

together and evaluation of existing hospice research, evaluations, and information pertaining to hospices in this country and abroad. Hospice health-policy analysis attempts to articulate and provide evidence for the pros and cons of alternative options or strategies facing a decision maker in the hospice arena. Policy analysis should rarely be based on a single program evaluation; it ideally should be a synthesis of programmatic evaluation as well as a review of relevant nonexperimental and experimental research on specific and sensitive hospice issues.

## Why Evaluate Hospice?

Hospice programs in the United States should be evaluated for the reasons listed below:

1. To demonstrate to other groups that the hospice program is an effective health care program.
2. To justify past or projected expenditures.
3. To determine costs.
4. To gain support for expansion of facilities.
5. To determine future objectives.
6. To determine program efficiency.

In summary, from the hospice administrator or planner perspective, program evaluation helps to answer basic questions about whether the program is good and whether it helps ensure accountability by administrators, staff, patients, and families. Evaluations should help keep the hospice emphasis on end results and should help promote training of staff.

A number of recently identified developments have focused much attention on hospice program evaluation. Among these are: 1) the growing involvement of federal government in hospice services with respect to financing and provision, 2) growing demands for public accountability, and 3) community involvement (financial and social) in rendering hospice services.

The reasons for evaluating a specific hospice program will differ depending on the interested parties. The perspectives of the hospice agency, hospice administrator, and funding agency, public or patient groups, and the evaluator are likely to differ in varying degrees about: 1) the objectives to be evaluated; 2) the types of evaluation that need to be conducted; 3) the research design that needs to be employed; 4) the relevant measures of program input, process, and impact; 5) the collection of the data; 6) the analysis of the data; and 7) the inferences drawn about the data.

## The Evaluation Process

The hospice program evaluation process can be subdivided into three basic categories. The first pertains to the exact specification of program objectives and concerns itself with the program planning stage. The second category pertains to the organization of resources to carry out the hospice program. This can also be considered the program implementation stage. The third, final, and probably most significant stage is the assessment of program performance, which may otherwise be called the program impact stage. Figure 8–1 should clarify these three important areas.

The specification of objectives is the most crucial aspect of any beginning or developing organization. Every organization must have written goals and objectives or it cannot be understood, implemented, or evaluated.

The nature and content of the objectives must be carefully respectful of the overall goals of the hospice organization. Priorities must be set for the objectives of the hospice program, in harmony with the target population that it intends to serve. Each specific objective must be given a place in the hospice organization in order of importance, for each hospice program will have a multiplicity of specific program objectives. It must be understood that not all objectives can be scientifically evaluated.

## Use of the Scientific Method in the Evaluation Procedure

It is strongly recommended that use of the scientific method in performing hospice program evaluation be considered by administration. It must be understood that use of the scientific method in performing such an evaluation requires considerable forethought as well as scrupulous attention to detail. Before an evaluation can take place, hospice program objectives must be identified and translated into measurable terms. Recognition of the problems with which the program must cope is advised, lest the exigencies of program development invalidate an ongoing, inflexible course of evaluation. A specific and sensitive data retrieval system must be developed and utilized. Program activities should be profiled and standardized to facilitate measurement of changes that take place.

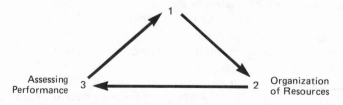

**Figure 8–1** Setting Program Objectives for Evaluation of Hospice

Measures used to monitor effectiveness of program activities should have proven reliability and validity. Where changes are detected, the possibility that they may be due to some factor other than the activity of the hospice program should be considered. Those effects attributable to the work of the program should be rated for durability and generalizability. Progress in evaluation of terminal care services should be made as a function of the use of the scientific method—the examination of specific program objectives and their attendant assumptions, the development of measurable criteria explicitly related to those specific objectives, and the controlled determination of the extent to which the objectives are met. These criteria characterize true evaluation research as distinct from subjective assessment or anecdotal reports which so predominantly characterize most hospice program evaluation.

An evaluation of a hospice program should accomplish even more than discovery of whether and to what extent objectives have been met. An evaluation can pinpoint causes of specific successes and failures and aid in directing the program administrators toward formulas for success.

Practical problems of adhering to principles of research, in opposition to administrative considerations, constitute a greater challenge to execution of an evaluative study than do the rigors of those principles. Principles of research dictate that specific rather than entire programs should be measured, that methods and objectives of terminal care programs should be clearly defined, and that control groups should be used as a basis for comparison. However, the nature of most social service programs works against application of experimental methodology. Service personnel, although highly qualified for delivery of terminal care, usually lack training or skills necessary for evaluative research. Their collection and interpretation of data is likely to be unsophisticated and suffer from the lack of strict scientific guidance. Furthermore, the irregularity with which scientific standards are adhered to by various staff members results in collection of unreliable data. Attempts at self-evaluation by terminal care programs both incorporate problems of ill-prepared personnel and inevitably preclude objectivity. Personal bias is unavoidable when funding or reputation of one's program is at stake. In addition, the need to carry out self-evaluation as well as usual service activities prevents allocation of sufficient time, money, and personnel for planning, collection of data, and analysis. Unfortunately, administrative resistance and barriers, lack of resources, and failure to utilize findings frequently operate against objective evaluation, which is the preferable alternative to self-evaluation.

In terms of administrative relationships, even assuming the most favorable interpersonal relationships, the program evaluation team is bound to be at odds to some degree with the action team from start to finish. This organizational tension arises from a number of factors, including philosophical differences, competition for resources, the tremen-

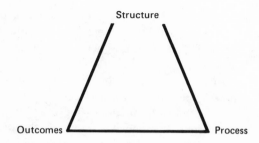

**Figure 8–2** A Structure for Evaluation

dous burden that proper evaluation places on the conduct of the program being evaluated, the special role of the evaluator, and differences in professional values.

In the event of administrative cooperation, the subject matter may pose problems for evaluation of facilities for terminal care. Arbitrary selection of target problems stresses traditional activities at the expense of developing areas. Evaluation of facilities and resources is too frequently emphasized while effectiveness of interventions is too often ignored. The Donabedian (1966) model of evaluation research proposes an appealing solution to substitution of facilities and activities for achievement. Donabedian perceives resources and effort expended as matters of importance in characterization of program rather than assessment of program effectiveness. He has outlined a structure for evaluation (see Figure 8–2) that points to three components—structure, process, and outcome—as the basis of evaluation.

Measurement of outcomes allows determination of program effectiveness, and description of structure and process provides the basis for assumptions of causality. Program goals and objectives are the dependent variables of such an evaluation. One must be able to put the specific program objectives into testable hypotheses.

## Methods in Collecting Evaluation Data

One can collect evaluation information in a variety of ways, including:

1. Written self-report measures.
2. Observations.
3. Interviews.
4. Performance tests.
5. Record reviews.
6. Written tests of ability or knowledge.

## 1. WRITTEN SELF-REPORT MEASURES

Written self-report measures ask people to tell about their attitudes, beliefs, feelings, and perceptions. Questionnaires, rating and ranking scales, the Semantic Differential, the Q-sort, and diaries are among the techniques most frequently used in program evaluation.

*Questionnaires* are self-administered survey forms that consist of a set of questions. Answers to questionnaire items can require free responses (short answers), or they can be structured into "forced" choices (multiple-choice items). Questionnaires are frequently used in large-scale evaluations to obtain participants' reactions and opinions. They are less expensive to construct than most measures; but the kind of information available from them is limited, and people don't always answer the questions truthfully.

*Rating scales* can be used for self-assessment or for appraisals of other people, groups, events, or products. For example, the efficiency of the new appointment system can be rated on a five-point scale from one for not very efficient to five for very efficient. Rating scales are particularly useful to reduce judgmental data to a manageable form. They are relatively easy to complete, and they produce relatively objective data.

Unfortunately, they are subject to many types of bias—some raters are lenient and others are not, and sometimes raters let their personal feelings influence their ratings (called a halo effect). Further, the amount of information obtainable from rating scales is limited because the rating categories are never perfect.

*Ranking scales* involve putting a set of items into a hierarchy according to some value or preference. Asking a pharmacist to rank four drugs from one to four according to their potency in treating headaches is an example. Like rating scales, ranking scales are easy to complete and produce objectified data. But rank ordering involves dealing with a long list of items and takes a lot of time. Ranking scales sometimes ask people to make distinctions they can't really see.

*Semantic differential* is used to measure attitudes by relying on the indirect meanings of words. For example, parents of pediatric patients might be asked to rate their child's physician by using a series of seven-point scales like the following:

| | | | | | | | |
|---|---|---|---|---|---|---|---|
| Caring | ____ | ____ | ____ | ____ | ____ | ____ | ____ Unconcerned |
| Rushed | ____ | ____ | ____ | ____ | ____ | ____ | ____ Relaxed |
| Pleasant | ____ | ____ | ____ | ____ | ____ | ____ | ____ Disagreeable |
| Confident | ____ | ____ | ____ | ____ | ____ | ____ | ____ Inexperienced |

The Semantic Differential is relatively easy to complete, it produces objectified data, and respondents usually find it harder to choose "socially acceptable" answers than when they use an ordinary rating scale, but it can be quite difficult to score.

The *Q-sort* requires individuals to place a series of items or statements into rating categories so that some minimum number of items is assigned to each category. For example, nursing educators could be asked to rate ten textbooks as "above average" or "below average" so that at least two texts are assigned to each category (the remaining texts can be rated either way). In this case, no average category was permitted.

Q-sorts produce objectified data, and they force respondents to establish priorities among items that are being compared in an evaluation. But the Q-sort requires people to make very difficult distinctions, the directions are often hard to follow, and the resulting data can require complex analysis methods.

*Diary techniques* ask people to keep daily or weekly accounts of specific behaviors, attitudes, thoughts, or events. The *critical incident* technique asks people to record only those things that are particularly important, unique, useful, or revelatory. For example, outpatients might be asked to keep a diary for two months describing difficulties they encountered because of their asthma.

Diaries and critical incidents permit people to describe unique situations in their own words; but people sometimes forget to maintain them, and they are often difficult to score and interpret.

## 2. Observations

Another information collection technique frequently used in evaluations is an eyewitness account of individual behavior or program activities. Observations of the number of patients reading the medical literature available in a waiting room might be made, for example, as an indication of the materials' usefulness. The information collected by observers can be reported by checklists, rating scales, field notes, and summary reports.

*Standardized observations* require careful planning so that the information obtained is accurate. Observations can give information collectors firsthand information about a program, and they are often the only feasible and economical way to gather certain kinds of information. But it is costly to train observers, and several may be needed to get reliable results. Another drawback is that people who know they are being observed may not behave normally.

*Time-sampling observations* involve repeated observations of a given situation. For example, observers may note which participants in a continuing medical education program ask questions during ten consecutive five-minute intervals.

Time sampling allows firsthand observations of a program, and the many observations make it possible to identify unusual events that might otherwise be viewed as routine occurrences. When all the observations are made one after the other, however, they are likely to depict only one particular situation and not the program as a whole.

### 3. INTERVIEWS

An interview is an information collection technique in which one person talks to another or to a group. Interviews can be completely unstructured and spontaneous, or may include only questions determined ahead of time. If you use multiple-choice questions, even the response categories are predetermined.

*Face-to-face interviews* may be used, for example, to find out why participants dropped out of a program and might consist of three basic questions with a series of two or more in-depth questions for each basic question asked. The best thing about the face-to-face interview is that it permits probing of sensitive subjects like attitudes or values. However, interviews are usually time-consuming and expensive, and interviewers must be given special training.

*Telephone interviews* also permit in-depth probing of sensitive issues and are less costly than face-to-face interviews. However, they are still expensive when compared to questionnaires. Because not everyone has a telephone and because some people are reluctant to reveal their feelings or give personal information over the phone, such interviews have definite limitations.

### 4. PERFORMANCE TESTS

*Performance tests* require people to complete a task or make something, and then the quality of the performance or product is assessed. One example of a performance test is videotaping an interview between a psychiatrist and a patient and then having experts view the tape and rate the interviewer's skills using a specially designed scale.

The major advantage of performance testing is that it relies on tasks that are close to "real world" activities. It is often very time-consuming and expensive, however, because performance tests generally have to be administered individually, and they sometimes require the use of special equipment.

### 5. RECORD REVIEWS

Record reviews involve collecting evaluation information by going through program-related documents. In a weight reduction program, for example, attendance records might be reviewed to see if participants regularly came to group sessions, and medical records might be reviewed to find out about weight loss.

Record reviews are "unobtrusive" in the sense that they do not interfere with the activities of the program being evaluated. They can also be relatively inexpensive because no new data collection is required. One problem is that program documents may be disorganized, unavailable, or incomplete.

### 6. Written Tests of Ability or Knowledge

Written achievement tests are among the most commonly used measurement techniques.

*Achievement tests* measure competency in a given subject. They can be developed by the program or evaluation staff or be bought from publishers. Achievement tests can be used to measure a diverse range of factors from knowledge of anatomy to skill in taking a patient's history.

The advantages of achievement tests are that they can be administered to large groups at relatively low cost and that carefully developed and validated tests are available in many subject areas.

One disadvantage is that achievement tests must be properly validated to provide accurate information, and this can be a costly procedure. Another is that having high scores on a test of factual knowledge doesn't always mean that the individual can apply that knowledge.

### Summary

Evaluation can be viewed as an independent check on the adequacy of hospice program planning. On the other hand, evaluation will contribute to the planning phase of program development by delineating problems, resources, and objectives, and by determining rational courses of action. True evaluation research allows determination of the extent to which stated program objectives are met through program activities.

Roos (1973) notes that it will be increasingly important in future years to fit program evaluation research strategies to the specific nature of the program under study and the types of decisions to be made. Programs with clearly defined goals and objectives, where it is possible to obtain a high degree of knowledge, are appropriate for experimental and quasi-experimental designs. In contrast, programs that have ill-defined goals, that are in their beginning stages, and that show a low degree of obtainable knowledge are more appropriate for process-oriented evaluations.

Program evaluations, of both a process- and outcome-oriented nature,

**Table 8–1**   Advantages and Disadvantages of Evaluation Techniques

| Information Collection Methods | | Advantages | Disadvantages |
|---|---|---|---|
| Observations | Standard Observations | Can observe events firsthand | Observers can change the environment<br>Inter- and intra-observer reliability can be difficult to obtain |
| | Time-Sampling Observations | Can observe events firsthand<br>More opportunities to observe | Observers can change the environment<br>Inter- and intra-observer reliability can be difficult to obtain |
| Interviews | Face-to-Face Interviews | Permits in-depth probing<br>Sensitive issues can be discussed | Costly<br>Inter- and intra-rater reliability can be difficult to obtain |
| | Telephone | Permits in-depth probing<br>Sensitive issues can be discussed<br>Less costly than face-to-face interviews | Costly<br>Some people may not have telephones<br>More difficult to probe or discuss sensitive issues |
| Performance Tests | | Close to real-world situations | Costly<br>Generally must be administered individually<br>Can require special equipment or apparatus |
| Record Review | | Unobtrusive<br>Can be inexpensive<br>No new data collection required | Documents may be disorganized or unavailable |
| Written Tests of Ability | Achievement Tests | Can be administered to large groups at relatively low costs<br>Many published, standardized tests are available | Expensive to develop and validate<br>High scores do not necessarily imply that the tested knowledge can be applied |

**Table 8–1**   *continued*

| Information Collection Methods | | Advantages | Disadvantages |
|---|---|---|---|
| Written Self-Report Measures | Questionnaires | Can be administered to large groups at relatively low costs | Can be difficult to obtain sensitive information<br>Respondents may not always be truthful<br>Must follow up to obtain adequate numbers of respondents |
| | Rating Scales | Easy to complete<br>Produces objectified data<br>Reduces judgmental data into a manageable form | Responses may be biased because some raters are lenient and others are strict<br>Amount of information obtainable is circumscribed by the rating categories<br>Halo effect |
| | Ranking Scales | Easy to complete<br>Produces objectified data | Difficult to rank a long list of items<br>Distinctions are called for that are not perceived |
| | Semantic Differences | Easy to complete<br>Produces objectified data<br>More difficult to give "socially acceptable" responses | Difficult to score |
| | Q-Sorts | Produces objectified data<br>Forces respondents to establish priorities among items | Distinctions are called for that are not perceived<br>Directions can be too elaborate<br>Can require complex data-analysis method |
| | Diaries and Critical Incidents | Permits people to describe unique situations in their own words | People don't maintain them<br>Difficult to score and interpret |

can be expected to continue to grow. Program administrators, providers, planners, evaluation researchers, and policy makers will need to become increasingly sophisticated about the problems and issues involved in assessing social service and health care programs. This ranges from being better able to specify program objectives, components, and categories of evaluation, to the consideration of alternative research designs, data-collection systems, assessment of the reliability and validity of measures, appropriate choice of data analysis, and increased competence in making sure that the results of the program evaluation are useful to the decision makers for whom they are intended and are used by them.

There is an increased need under the hospice umbrella for training health professionals of *all* categories and exposing them to some basic considerations involved in the evaluation of hospice programs. Hospice health care professionals will need to have a common understanding of the basic issues in assessing programs and be able to speak a common language. As hospice personnel participate in evaluation activities, hospice health care professionals may also learn more about themselves, in addition to the hospice program. Such self-discovery can contribute to increased personal and professional growth.

# 9

*Conclusion*

HOSPICE CARE in the United States is relatively new; the first hospice home-care program was offered by Hospice, Inc. of New Haven, Connecticut, in 1974. But was it new? And if so, what about it was different from home care for dying persons or care of people in the established United States health care system?

It can be argued that there is nothing new in hospice. Care of dying persons was, in fact, offered by Calvary Hospital in New York City before hospice arrived. Brompton's formula for pain control was in use before the contemporary hospice movement. Spiritual healing has been one aspect of religious life for many years, and comprehensive delivery of health care sources has been a professed goal of our health care long before hospice.

But somewhere, over some extended period of time, something went askew. The simple became more complex, and with the complexity of American living, especially in health care, there was a loss of humanism, a loss of the kindness of human touching and caring.

Hospice has intruded into the spiral of health care technology with startling impact. It has not been the newness of hospice, but rather its challenge to the humanness of health care that has disturbed the status quo. Hospice has advocated for the quality of life, for living until death, for the absence of pain, for the maintenance of personal control, for the maintenance of the family. Hospice is being folded into a larger philosophical framework in which there is renewed recognition that emotional well-being is at least as important as physical health (Holden, 1979).

But what the contemporary hospice movement has shown us is that there is a specific mixture of philosophy, services, staff, and community which, when put together in the right combination, can be more effective than prior methods of providing care for dying persons. This combination of services is hospice care. Hospice care has a definition, a content, an expected style of service, and an organizational integrity. Hospice does exist in our health care system; but as soon as it was established, the debate began regarding its life expectancy.

There is current recognition that hospice care must be closely related to the mainstream of health care activity in order to exist and have maximum impact on care of the dying person, not only to avoid the "house of death" stigma, but also to make an important statement regarding the direction health care as a whole should take.

At present, "cure" and "care" are seen as two radically different modes for the health professional—the one oriented toward aggressive physical measures to save and prolong life, the other toward easing the way to the inevitable. However, as Lorenz K. Y. Ng of the National Institute of Mental Health has said, this apparent dichotomy (the Cartesian duality that has been hanging around our necks for three hundred years) could be resolved if the focus of all medical care were on furthering "wellness"— physical, emotional, social, and spiritual. Thus the hospice movement, far from being a separate and specialized phenomenon, supplies a model for getting the whole health system back on the track (Holden, 1979).

How long will hospice be necessary? For as long as people die.

# References

## Chapter 1

AGICH, G. "The Ethics of Terminal Care," *Death Education* 2 (Spring/Summer 1978): 163–171.

BERKI, S., and HESTON, A. "Introduction," *The Annals* 399, January 1972, pp. v–x.

BRADY, E. M. "Telling the Story: Ethics and Aging," in Catholic Hospital Association, *Major Addresses of the Institutes on Hospices*. St. Louis: Catholic Hospital Association, 1978.

BROWN, E. L. *Newer Dimensions of Patient Care*. New York: Russell Sage Foundation, 1961.

FEIFEL, H. *The Meaning of Death*. New York: McGraw-Hill, 1959.

———. 1977. *New Meanings of Death*. New York: McGraw-Hill.

FOSTER, Z., WALD, F., and WALD, H. "The Hospice Movement: A Backward Glance at Its First Two Decades." *The New Physician*, May 1978, 17, pp. 21–24.

FULTON, R., ed. *Death and Identity*. Bowie, Md.: Charles Press, 1976.

GARFIELD, C. *Psychosocial Care of the Dying Patient*. New York: McGraw-Hill, 1978.

GLASER, B., and STRAUSS, A. *Awareness of Dying*. Chicago: Aldine, 1965.

General Accounting Office. "Hospice Care—A Growing Concept in the United States." *Report to the Congress*, March 6, 1979, HRD–79–50.

HACKLEY, J. "Full Service Hospice Offers Home, Day and Inpatient Care." *Hospitals*, November 1, 1977, pp. 84–87.

KALISH, R. "Death and Dying in a Social Context." In *Handbook of Aging and the Social Sciences*, R. Binstock and E. Shanas, eds. New York: Van Nostrand Reinhold, 1976.

KASTENBAUM, R. *Death, Society and Human Experience*. St. Louis: C. V. Mosby, 1977.

KÜBLER-ROSS, E. *On Death and Dying*. New York: MacMillan Co., 1969.

LACK, S. "New Haven (1974), Characteristics of a Hospice Program of Care." *Death Education* 2 (Spring/Summer, 1978): 41–52.

LAMERS, W. "Marin County (1976), Development of Hospice of Marin." *Death Education* 2 (Spring/Summer, 1978): 53–62.

MECHANIC, D. "Human Problems and the Organization of Health Care." *The Annals,* January 1972, pp. 1–11.

National Hospice Organization. *Hospice Principles and Standards,* February 23, 1979.

ROSSMAN, I., and KISSICK, W. "Home Care and the Cancer Patient." In *American Cancer Society, The Physician and the Total Care of the Cancer Patient.* New York: The American Cancer Society, 1962.

SAUNDERS, C. "Dying They Live: St. Christopher's Hospice." In *New Meanings of Death.* H. Feifel, ed. New York: McGraw-Hill, 1977.

SCHNEIDMAN, E., ed. *Death: Current Perspectives.* Palo Alto, Calif.: Mayfield, 1976.

SOMERS, A. "The Nation's Health: Issues for the Future." *The Annals,* January 1972, pp. 160–174.

STODDARD, S. *The Hospice Movement.* Briarcliff Manor, N.Y.: Stein and Day, 1978.

WEISMAN, A. *The Realization of Death: A Guide for Psychological Autopsy.* New York: Jason Aronson, 1974.

WILSON, D., AJEMIAN, I., and MOUNT, B. "Montreal (1975), The Royal Victoria Hospital Palliative Care Service." *Death Education* 2 (Spring/Summer 1978): 3–19.

## Chapter 2

*American Journal of Nursing.* January 1975, p. 99.

DAVIDSON, G. "In Search of Models of Care." *Death Education* 2 (Spring/Summer 1978): 145–161.

LEICH, T. "To Comfort Always." In *Major Addresses on the Institutes on Hospices.* St. Louis: Catholic Hospital Association, 1978.

MARLOW, D. *Textbook of Pediatric Nursing.* Philadelphia: W. B. Saunders, 1977.

MARTINSON, I. "Why Don't We Let Them Die at Home?" *RN,* January 1976, pp. 53–65.

―――. Personal Conversation. March, 1979.

MARTINSON, I., GRIS, D., ANGLEN, M., PETERSON, E., NESBIT, M., and KERSEY, J. "Home Care for the Dying Child." *American Journal of Nursing* 77 (November 1977): 1815–1817.

MOUSTAKAS, C. *Creative Life.* New York: D. Van Nostrand, 1977, p. 1.

SAUNDERS, C. "Watch with Me." *Nursing Times* 61, November 1965.

SCIPIEN, G., BARNARD, M., CHARD, M., HOWE, J., PHILLIPS, P. *Comprehensive Pediatric Nursing.* New York: McGraw-Hill, 1975.

## Chapter 3

BAINES, M., ed. *Drug Control of Common Symptoms.* St. Christopher's Hospice, n.d.

BENOLIEL, J., and CROWLEY, D. *The Pain in Pain: New Concepts.* American Cancer Society Professional Education Publication, 1974.

DAVITZ, L., SAMESHINA, Y., and DAVITZ, J. "Suffering as Viewed in Six Different Cultures." *American Journal of Nursing* 76 (August 1976): 1296–1297.

FARR, W. "Oral Morphine for Control of Pain in Terminal Cancer." *Arizona Medicine* 35 (March 1978): 167–170.

LACK, S. "New Haven (1974), Characteristics of a Hospice Program of Care." *Death Education* 1 (Spring/Summer 1978): 41–52.

LAMERS, W. In "Marin Hospice: Answering the Prayers of the Terminally Ill," E. Rubin. *Mill Valley Record,* May 4, 1977.

LAMERTON, R. Lecture at Hillhaven Hospice, Tucson, Arizona, April 1977.

McKORKLE, R., and YOUNG, K. "Development of a Symptom Distress Scale." *Cancer Nursing,* October 1978.

MARTINSON, I., GRIS, D., ANGLEN, M., PETERSON, E., NESBIT, M., and KERSEY, J. "Home Care for the Dying Child." *American Journal of Nursing* 77 (November 1977): 1815–1817.

MELZACK, R., OFIESH, J., and MOUNT, B. "The Bromptom's Mixture: Effects on Pain in Cancer Patients." *Canadian Medical Association Journal,* July 17 1976, pp. 125–128.

MOUNT, B., ADJAMIAN, I., and SCOTT, J. "Use of Bromptom's Mixture in Treating Chronic Pain in Malignant Disease." *Canadian Medical Association Journal,* July 17, 1976, pp. 122–124.

PARKES, C. "Evaluation of Family Care in Terminal Illness." In *The Family and Death,* E. Pritchard et al., eds. New York: Columbia University Press, 1977.

SAUNDERS, C. "Control of Pain in Terminal Cancer," *Nursing Times,* July 22, 1976, pp. 1133–1135.

——, 1978. "Patient Care: An Introduction," in *Topics in Therapeutics,* D. W. Vere, ed. London: Pitman Medical Pub. Co. Ltd.

SHANFIELD, S., and KILLINGSWORTH, R. "The Psychiatric Aspect of Pain." *Psychiatric Annals* 7 (January 1977): 24–35.

TWYCROSS, R. "The Use of Narcotic Analgesics in Terminal Illness." *Journal of Medical Ethics* 11 (November 1975): 10–17.

——. 1976. "The Measurement of Pain in Terminal Cancer." *Journal of International Medical Research* 4 (April 1976): 58–67.

VALENTINE, A., STECKEL, S., and WEINTRAUB, M. "Pain Relief for Cancer Patients." *American Journal of Nursing,* December 1978.

VERE, D. W. "Pharmacology of Morphine Drugs used in Terminal Care." In *Topics in Therapeutics,* D. W. Vere. London: Pitman Medical Pub. Co. Ltd., 1978.

## Chapter 4

CRAVEN, J., and WALD, F. "Hospice Care for Dying Patients." *American Journal of Nursing* 75 (October 1975): 1816–1822.

FEIFEL, H. *New Meanings of Death.* New York: McGraw-Hill, 1977.

FULTON, R., ed. *Death and Identity.* Bowie, Md.: Charles Press, 1976.

# 178  *References*

MILLER, I., and SOLOMON, R. "The Development of Group Services for the Elderly." In *Social Work Practice: People and Environments,* C. Germain. New York: Columbia University Press, 1979.

PARKS, K. M. *Bereavement.* Markham, Ontario: Penguin Books, 1972.

ROGERS, B. "Using the Creative Process with the Terminally Ill." *Death Education* 2 (Spring/Summer 1978): 123–126.

## Chapter 5

FEIFEL, H. "The Taboo on Death." *American Behavioral Science,* 1963.

———. 1977. *New Meaning of Death.* New York: McGraw-Hill.

HARPER, B. *Death: The Coping Mechanism of the Health Professional.* Greenville, S. C.: Southeastern University Press, 1977.

LACK, S. and BUCKINGHAM, R. *First American Hospice.* New Haven, Conn.: Hospice Inc., 1978.

LAMERTON, R. *Care of the Dying.* Hackney, England: Priority Press Ltd., 1973.

MASLACK, C. "Burned-Out." *Human Behavior* 5 (September 1976): 16–22.

PINES, A., and MASLACK, C. "Characteristics of Staff Burnout in Mental Health Settings." *Hospital and Community Psychiatry* 29 (April 1973): 233–237.

STEINFELD, J. "Introduction." In *Death: The Coping Mechanism of the Health Professional,* B. Harper. Greenville, S. C.: Southeastern University Press, 1977.

## Chapter 6

CHAN, L. "Hospice: A New Building Type to Comfort the Dying." *American Institute of Architects Journal,* December 1976, pp. 42–45.

ITTELSON, W. In *Environmental Psychology: Man and his Physical Setting,* Roshansky, H., Ittelson, W., and Revlin, L., eds. New York: Holt, Rinehart and Winston, 1970.

THOMPSON, J., and GOLDIN, G. *The Hospital: A Social and Architectural History.* New Haven, Conn.: Yale University Press, 1975.

## Chapter 7

ENGLISH, D. "Can Hospice Be Accomplished Financially?" In *Major Addresses of the Institutes on Hospices.* St. Louis: Catholic Hospital Association, 1978.

GIBSON. M. "How Can It Be Accomplished Financially?" In *Major Addresses of the Institutes on Hospices.* St. Louis: Catholic Hospital Association, 1978.

HACKLEY, J. "Financing and Accrediting Hospices," *Hospital Progress,* March 1979. pp. 51–53.

LACK, S, and BUCKINGHAM, R. *First American Hospice.* New Haven, Conn.: Hospice Inc., 1978.

REICH, W. "Ethical Issues Relating to Research Involving Elderly Subjects." *The Gerontologist* 18 (August 1978): 326–337.


## Chapter 8

DONABEDIAN, A. "Evaluating the Quality of Medical Care." *Milbank Memorial Fund Quarterly* 44 (1966): 166–203.

ROOS, N. P. "Evaluation, Quasi-experimentation, and Public Policy: Observations by a Short-term Bureaucrat." In *Quasi-experimental Testing Theory and Evaluation Policy,* Caporaso, J., and Roos, L. L., Jr., eds. Chicago: Northwestern University Press, 1973.


## Chapter 9

HOLDEN, C. "Pain, Dying, and the Health Care System." *Science* 203 (March 1979): 984–985.

# Bibliography

ABBOTT, JOHN W. "Hospice." *Aging Magazine,* November/December 1978, p. 38.

ABRAMS, RUTH. "The Patient with Cancer—His Changing Pattern of Communication." *New England Journal of Medicine* 274, no. 6 (February 10, 1966): 317–22.

AGICH, GEORGE J. "The Ethics of Terminal Care." *Death Education* 2, no. 1–2 (Spring/Summer 1978): 163–71.

AJEMIAN, INA. "An Oral Morphine Mixture for Intractable Pain." *Canadian Family Physician,* 23, no. 1500 (1977).

———. "The Royal Victoria Hospital Palliative Care Service." *Death Education* 2, no. 1–2 (Spring/Summer 1978): 3–39.

ALSOFROM, J. "Hospice Way of Dying at Home with Friends and Family." *American Medical News* 8, February 21, 1977, pp. 7–9.

AMES, RICHARD P.; MINEAU, DAVID; and PETRUSHEVICH, KATHY. "Mercy Hospice: A Hospital-based Program." *Hospital Progress,* March 1979, pp. 63–67.

"Assumptions and Principles Underlying Standards for Terminal Care." *The International Work Group in Death, Dying and Bereavement,* January 3, 1978.

BANKS, LEO. "Hillhaven Hospice: The Last Stop." *Tucson Magazine,* November 1977, pp. 34–38.

BARDEN, J. C. "Calvary Gives Terminal Patients an Integrated Approach to Death." Reprinted from The *New York Times,* distributed by Calvary Hospice.

BARNARD, CHARLES N. "Good Death." *Family Health* 5 (April 1973): 40–42.

BARTLETT, LINDA. "Love, the Final Act of Life." *Washington Post,* April 24, 1977.

BAUMAN, REV. EDWARD. "Coming to Terms with Death." *Aging Magazine,* November/December 1978, p. 6.

BECKER, ERNEST. *The Denial of Death.* New York: The Free Press, 1973.

BENOLIEL, JEANNE Q. "Talking to Patients About Death." *Nursing Forum* 9, no. 3 (1970): 255–69.

BERDES, CELIA. *Social Services for the Aged, Dying & Bereaved in International Perspective.* Washington, D.C.: International Federation on Aging, 1978.

"A Better Way of Dying." *Time,* June 5, 1978, p. 66.

Blue Cross Association and Blue Shield Association. *Initial Statement on Hospice Care and Payment for Hospice Services,* approved November 8, 1978 by Board of Blue Cross and Blue Shield Associations.

BRADY, E. MICHAEL. "Telling the Story: Ethics and Dying." *Hospital Progress,* March 1979, pp. 57–62.

BRAUN, HOWARD and GILARDI, DENNIS. "The Hospice Concept." *L & H Perspective,* Fall/Winter 1978, pp. 36–37.

BREINDEL, CHARLES L., and BOYLE, RUSSELL M. "Implementing a Multi-phased Hospice Program." *Hospital Progress,* March 1979, pp. 42–45.

BRIM, O. G. *The Dying Patient.* New York: Russell Sage, 1970.

BUCKINGHAM, ROBERT W., III. "A Guide to Evaluation Research in Terminal Care Programs." *Death Education* 2, no. 1–2 (Spring/Summer 1978): 127–41.

———. "Living With the Dying: Use of the Technique of Participant Observation." *Canadian Medical Association Journal* 115, no. 12 (December 18, 1976): 1211–15.

BUCKINGHAM, ROBERT; KRON, JOAN; and WALD, HENRY. *The Hospice Concept.* New York: New York Health Sciences Publishing Corporation, 1977.

BURTON, REP. JOHN L. "The Human Value of the Hospice Program." *Congressional Record,* July 31, 1978, pp. E4176–77.

CALIFANO, JOSEPH A., JR. "Remarks of Secretary Joseph A. Califano, Jr., Department of Health, Education, and Welfare to the National Hospice Organization First Annual Congress." *HEW News Press Release,* October 5, 1978.

———. "Secretary Califano Pledges Support for Hospice Movement." *Aging Magazine,* November/December 1978, p. 20.

"Care of the Dying." Symposium at Royal College of Physicians with Sheila Hancock, Cicely Saunders, W. F. Anderson, E. Wilkes, Sir David Smithers, Ronald Gibson, M. P. Daniel, J. McTrustry, B. J. McNutty, W. Mitchell, K. R. O. Porter. *British Medical Journal,* January 6, 1973, pp. 29–43.

CAREY, R., and POSAUAC, E. "Attitudes of Physicians on Disclosing Information to and Maintaining Life for Terminal Patients." *Omega* 9, no. 1 (1978–79): 67–71.

CARPENTER, JAMES and WYLIE, CHARLES. "On Aging, Dying, and Denying." *Public Health Reports* 89, no. 5 (September/October 1974): 403–7.

CASSELL, E. J. "Learning to Die." *Bulletin—N.Y. Academy of Medicine* 49, no. 12 (1973): 1110–18.

Catholic Hospital Association. *Major Addresses of the Institutes on Hospice.* St. Louis: Catholic Hospital Association, 1978.

CHAN, LO-YI. "Hospice: A New Building Type to Comfort the Dying." *AIA Journal,* December 1976, pp. 42–45.

"Characteristics of a Hospice Program and Assumptions and Principles of Care for the Terminally Ill." Prepared by *Second International Work Group Conference on Death, Dying and Bereavement,* distributed by Hospice of Marin, Kanfield, Ca., June, 1976.

CHARLES, ELEANOR. "A Hospice for the Terminally Ill." *New York Times,* March 13, 1977, 10:3.

"The Child Will Always Be There, Real Love Doesn't Die." *Psychology Today,* September 1976, pp. 48–52.

"Christmas at St. Christopher's." *American Journal of Nursing* 71, no. 12 (December 1971): 2325–27.

CLINES, FRANCIS X. "About New York: Waiting for the Blossoms of Spring in the Dusk of Life." *New York Times,* March 6, 1979.

COHEN, KENNETH P. *Hospice: Prescription for Terminal Care.* Germantown, Md.: Aspen Systems Corporation, 1979.

———. "A Study of the Hospice Movement in the United States and Canada: Legislation Survey Summary." Ph.D. dissertation, California Western University, January 1978.

COLEN, B. D. "Califano Backs Plan to Give Funds to Hospice Movement." *Washington Post,* October 5, 1978, A3.

———. "Nurse Speciality: Care for the Dying." *Washington Post,* August 24, 1975, A1–4.

CORBETT, TERRY L., and HAI, DOROTHY M. "Searching for Euthanatos: The Hospice Alternative." *Hospital Progress,* March 1979, pp. 38–41.

COSTA, PAUL T., JR., and KASTENBAUM, ROBERT. "Psychological Perspective on Death." *Annual Review of Psychology* 28 (1977): 225–49.

COTTER, ZITA M., SR. "Institutional Care of the Terminally Ill." *Hospital Progress* 52 (June 1971): 43–48.

COX, JAMES. "Springfield (1978)—St. John's Hospice." *Death Education* 2, no. 1–2 (Spring/Summer 1978): 83–95.

CRAVEN, J. "Hospice Care for Dying Patients." *American Journal of Nursing* 75 (1975): 1816–22.

DAVIDSON, GLEN W. *Hospice, Development & Administration.* Washington, D.C.: Hemisphere, 1978.

———. "In Search of Models of Care." *Death Education* 2 no. 1–2 (Spring/Summer 1978): 145–61.

DEFAREN, RUTH. "Hospices for the Dying." *The Humanist,* July/August 1974, pp. 28–29.

Department of Health, Education and Welfare, Health Care Financing Administration, Medicaid Hospice Projects. "Announcement of Projects." 1978.

Department of Health, Education and Welfare, Health Care Financing Administration. "Medicare and Medicaid Hospice Projects." 1978.

"A Dignified End to Living." *Yale Reports,* February 11, 1973.

DOBIHAL, E. F., JR. "Talk or Terminal Care." *Connecticut Medicine* 38 (1974): 145–61.

DOLE, SENATOR ROBERT. *Congressional Record,* May 18, 1978, S7689–90.

DOWNIE, P. A. "Havens of Peace." *Nursing Times* 69, no. 33 (August 16, 1973): 1068–70.

———. "A Personal Commentary on the Care of the Dying on the North American Continent." *Nursing Mirror* 139, no. 15 (October 10, 1974): 68–70.

DUNN, SISTER MARY KAYE. "A Philosophy For Living (The Hospice Program of Care)." New Haven, Conn.: Hospice, Inc.

EGERTON, ANN. "Building A Better Way to Die." *Baltimore Magazine,* April 1979.

ENGLISH, DAVID and WILSON, DOTTIE. "The Hospice Concept." Washington, D.C.: Elm Services, Inc., 1979.

ESPER, GEORGE. "Hospice Helps Patients to Live Until They Die; Families to Cope." *The Sunday Post—Closeup.* Reprinted by permission of the Bridgeport Post and Associated Press.

FARR, WILLIAM C. "Oral Morphine for Control of Pain in Terminal Cancer." *Arizona Medicine* 35, no. 3 (March 1978): 167–70.

FARR, WILLIAM C.; HACKLEY, JOHN; and MCINTIER, TERESA MARIE. "Tucson (1977)—Hillhaven Hospice." *Death Education* 2, no. 1–2 (Spring/Summer 1978): 63–82.

FATH, GERALD, REV. "Pastoral Care and the Hospice." *Hospital Progress,* March 1979, pp. 73, 35.

"Filling the Gap Between Home and Hospital: St. Anne's Hospice, England." *Nursing Mirror* 134, no. 5 (February 4, 1972).

"A Fix for Pain?" *Newsweek,* January 2, 1978, p. 41.

FOSTER, ZELDA; WALD, FLORENCE; and WALD, HENRY. "The Hospice Movement." *The New Physician* 27, no. 5 (May 1978): 21–24.

"Frequently Asked Questions About Hospice." New Haven, Conn.: Hospice, Inc., 1978.

FULTON, ROBERT. *Death, Grief, and Bereavement. A Bibliography: 1845–1975.* New York: Arno Press, 1977.

GARFIELD, CHARLES A. *Psychosocial Care of the Dying Patient.* New York: McGraw-Hill, 1977.

GARFIELD, C. A., and CLARK, R. O. "The Shanti Project: A Community Model." *Death Education* 1, no. 4 (Winter 1978): 397–408.

GARNER, JIM. "Palliative Care: It's Quality of Life Remaining that Matters." *Canadian Medical Association Journal* 115, no. 2 (July 17, 1976): 179–80.

GARRETT, DOROTHY N. "The Needs of the Seriously Ill and Their Families: The Haven Concept." *Aging Magazine,* November/December 1978, p. 12.

General Accounting Office. *Hospice Care—A Growing Concept in the U.S.* Washington, D.C.: U.S. Government Printing Office, March 6, 1979, HRD 79–50.

GOLEMAN, DANIEL. "We Are Breaking the Silence About Death." *Psychology Today,* September 1976, p. 44.

GOTTHEIL, EDWARD; McGURN, WEALTHA; and POLAK, OTTO. "Truth and/or Hope for the Dying Patient." *Nursing Digest,* March/April 1976, pp. 12–14.

GRAHAM, JORY. "A Time for Living, Home Provides Love, Sanctuary for the Dying." *Arizona Daily Star,* April 4, 1978.

GUREWITSCH, ELEANOR. "Calvary Hospital: The Newest Building, The Oldest Organization for the Terminally Ill." *Aging Magazine,* November/December 1978, p. 32.

GUSTAFSON, ELIZABETH. "Dying: The Career of the Nursing Home Patient." *Journal of Health and Social Behavior* 13 (September 1972): 226–34.

HACKETT, T. "Psychological Assistance for the Dying Patient and His Family." *Annual Review of Medicine,* 27, 1976.

HACKLEY, JOHN A. "Financing and Accrediting Hospices." *Hospital Progress,* March 1979, p. 51.

―――. "Full-Service Hospice Offers Home, Day and Inpatient Care." *Hospitals,* 2 (November 1, 1977).

―――. "How Can It Be Accomplished Financially?" Major Addresses of the Institutes on Hospices, sponsored by the Catholic Hospice Association, August 1978, pp. 1–23.

HALE, ELLEN. "Her Speciality is Death, But She Encourages New Life." *Tucson Citizen,* September 21, 1978.

HARPER, BERNICE CATHERINE. *The Coping Mechanism of the Health Professional.* Greenville, S.C.: Southeastern University Press, 1977.

HATFIELD, DAVID. "Tucson Hospice Profiled on CBS News Magazine." *Arizona Daily Star,* November 3, 1978.

HIGGINS, JAMES. "Up Out of the Valley of the Shadow of Death." *Arizona Daily Star,* December 17, 1977, p. 15.

Hillhaven Hospice. *Certificate of Need Application for Hillhaven Hospice Home Health Agency,* October 6, 1978, Tucson, Arizona.

Hillhaven Hospice. *Semi-Annual Report,* April 1, 1978–September 30, 1978, Tucson, Arizona.

"The Hospice Alternative: Sponsorship, Organizational, Financing, Accreditation, Pastoral, Ethical Issues." *Hospital Progress,* March 1979.

"The Hospice: An Alternative." *Journal of the American Medical Association* 236, no. 18 (November 1, 1976): 2047–48.

"Hospice . . . A Vision." New Haven, Conn.: New Haven Hospice, Inc., 1973.

"Hospice Care/Caring for the Terminally Ill." *The Blue Shield News,* February 1978.

"Hospice Care Growing in the United States, GAO Says." *Older American Reports,* March 21, 1979, p. 8.

"Hospice Care Helps People to Die Well." *New Horizons* 4, no. 2 (February 1979): 1–4. Publication of Eastern Nebraska Office on Aging.

"Hospice Family Centered Care for the Dying." *Cancer News* 32, no. 3 (Fall 1978): 10–13.

Hospice, Inc. *Application to the Connecticut State Council on Hospitals for the Endorsement of 44 Chronic Disease Hospital Beds for the Terminally Ill,* New Haven, Conn.

"The Hospice Movement." *Nursing Times* 72, no. 26 (July 1, 1976).

"Hospice New Trend in Health Care." *Long-Term Care Administration* 13, no. 1 (January 1, 1979). Published by American College of Nursing Home Administrators.

"Hospice Pilot Project." St. Luke's Hospital Center, New York, N.Y., November 1975.

HOLDEN, C. "Hospices: For the Dying, Relief from Pain and Fear." *Science* 193, no. 4251 (July 30, 1976): 389–91.

HOLFORD, J. M. "Terminal Care." *Nursing Times* 69, no. 4 (January 25, 1973): 113–16.

HOLLANDER, NEIL and EHRENFRIED, DAVID. "Reimbursing Hospice Care: A Blue Cross and Blue Shield Perspective." *Hospital Progress,* March 1979, pp. 54–55.

HUMPHREY, MURIEL. "The Hospice Movement." *Congressional Record*, May 25, 1978, S8367.

INGLES, T. "St. Christopher's Hospice." *Nursing Outlook* 22, no. 12 (December 1974): 759–63.

JACOBS, SELBY C., and OSTFELD, ADRIAN. "The Effects of Illness and Death of One Family Member on Other Family Members: A Review With Some Recommendations for Research and Medical Practice." In *Report of the Subcommittee on Terminal Illness*. Subcommittee on Terminal Illness, Department of Health, Education and Welfare, February 23, 1979.

JANETAKOS, JAMES D. "When the Patient Dies at Home." *Social Work* 23, no. 4 (July 1978).

JORDAN, LYETTE. "Hospice in America." *The Coevolution Quarterly* 14 (Summer 1977): 112–15.

KALISH, R. "Death and Dying in a Social Context." In *Handbook of Aging and the Social Sciences*, edited by R. Binstock and E. Shanas, New York: Van Nostrand Reinhold, 1976.

KASTENBAUM, ROBERT. "Dying, Innovations in Care." In *Death, Society and Human Experience*, ch. 13. Boston: C. V. Mosby Company, 1977.

———. ". . . Gone Tomorrow." *Geriatrics*, November 1974, pp. 127–34.

———. "On Death and Dying: Should We Have Mixed Feelings About Our Ambivalence Toward the Aged?" *Journal of Geriatric Psychiatry* 7, no. 1 (1974): 94–107.

———. "Time, Death and Ritual in Old Age." *The Study of Time* 2 (1975): 20–38.

KAVANAUGH, R. "Helping Patients Who Are Facing Death." *Nursing*, May 1974, pp. 35–41.

KELEMAN, STANLEY. *Living Your Dying*. New York: Random House, 1978.

KELLY, SISTER SIOBHAN. "Roncalli Home Care Hospice." *Major Addresses of the Institutes on Hospices*, sponsored by the Catholic Hospital Association, August 1978

KENNEDY, EDWARD. Press Release of the National Hospice Organization Meeting, Shoreham Hotel, Washington, D.C., October 5, 1978.

KERSTEIN, M. F. "Care for the Terminally Ill: A Hospice." *American Journal of Psychiatry* 129, no. 2 (August 1972): 237–38.

KILDUFF, MARSHALL. "Another Way to Treat the Dying." *San Francisco Chronicle*, April 10, 1975, p. 43.

KOFF, T. H. "Care of the Dying: An Experience in Living." *Journal of Long-Term Care Administration*, 1975.

———. "Social Rehearsal for Dying." *Journal of Long-Term Care Administration*, 1975.

KOHN, J. "Hospice Building Speaks on Many Emotional Levels to Patient, Family." *Modern Health Care* 6 (1976): 56–57.

———. "Hospice Movement Provides Human Alternative for Terminally Ill Patients." *Modern Health Care* 6 (1976): 26–28.

KRANT, MELVIN. "The Hospice Movement." *The New England Journal of Medicine* 299, no. 10 (September 7, 1978): 546–49.

———. "The Organized Care of the Dying Patient." *Hospital Practice*, January, 1972, pp. 101–8.

KRON, J. "Designing a Better Place to Die." *New York* 9 (1976): 43, 39.

KÜBLER-ROSS, E. "On Death and Dying." *Journal of American Medical Association* 221, no. 2 (July 10, 1972): 174–79. (Therapeutic Grand Rounds Number 36, with Stanford Wessler and Lewis V. Auidi.)

———. *To Live Until We Say Goodbye.* Englewood Cliffs, N.J.: Prentice-Hall, 1978.

KULIK, HOLIN. "Pain Assessment." Kaiser Foundation, Norwalk, Ca., January 1979.

LACK, SYLVIA A. "I Want to Die While I'm Still Alive." *Death Education* 1 (1977): 165–76.

———. "New Haven (1974)—Characteristics of a Hospice Program of Care." *Death Education* 2 no. 1–2. (Spring/Summer 1978): 41–52.

———. "Philosophy and Organization of a Hospice Program." In *Psychosocial Care of the Dying Patient,* edited by Charles A. Garfield. New York: McGraw-Hill, 1978, p. 79.

———. "The Hospice Concept—The Adult with Advanced Cancer." *Proceedings of American Cancer Society,* Second National Conference on Human Values and Cancer, 1977, pp. 160–66.

LACK, SYLVIA, and BUCKINGHAM, ROBERT. *First American Hospice: Three Years of Home Care.* New Haven: Hospice, Inc., 1978.

LACK, SYLVIA A., and LAMERTON, RICHARD. *The Hour Of Our Death.* London: MacMillan, 1974.

LAMERS, WILLIAM M. "Marin County (1976)—Development of Hospice of Marin." *Death Education* 2, no. 1–2 (Spring/Summer 1978): 53–62.

LAMERTON, RICHARD. *Care of the Dying.* London: Priory Press Ltd., 1973.

———. "Care of the Dying: Attitudes to Deathbed Nursing." *Nursing Times,* December 7, 1972, pp. 1544–45.

———. "Care of the Dying: Listening to the Dying." *Nursing Times,* January 4, 1973, p. 16.

———. "Care of the Dying: Religion and the Care of the Dying." *Nursing Times,* January 18, 1973, pp. 88–89.

———. "Care of the Dying: The Pains of Death." *Nursing Times,* January 11, 1973, pp. 56–57.

———. "Care of the Dying: Teamwork." *Nursing Times,* December 28, 1972, pp. 1642–43.

———. "Care of the Dying: The Right Time to Die." *Nursing Times,* December 14, 1972, p. 1578.

———. "Hospice: A Current Concept of Care for the Terminally Ill." Kenneth A. Hill Memorial Lecture, sponsored by Division of Social Perspective in Medicine, University of Arizona, 1955. Tape recording.

———. "The Need for Hospices." *Nursing Times,* January 23, 1975, pp. 155–58.

———. "Religion and the Care of the Dying." *Nursing Times,* January 18, 1973, pp. 88–89.

LEBLANG, THEODORE R. "Death with Dignity: A Tripartite Legal Response." *Death Education* 2, no. 1–2 (Spring/Summer 1978): 173–86.

LEICHT, THOMAS R. "To Comfort Always: The Hospice Alternative to the Care of Terminal Illness." Major Addresses of the Institutes on Hospices, August 1978. Sponsored by Catholic Hospital Association.

LE SHAN, L. "The World of the Patient in Severe Pain of Long Duration." *Journal of Chronic Diseases* 17, no. 1964: 119–26.

LIBMAN, JOAN. "Hospice Movement Stresses Family Care for the Terminally Ill." The *Wall Street Journal,* March 27, 1978, 1:1.

LIEGNER, L. M. "St. Christopher's Hospice, 1974." *Journal of American Medical Association* 234, no. 10 (December 8, 1975): 1047–48.

"Living with Dying." *Newsweek,* May 18, 1978, pp. 52–63.

LOONEY, J. F. "Hospice Care for the Adult." *American Journal of Nursing* 77, no. 11 (November 1977): 1812–15.

LUCIANO, LANI. "Hospice Care." *The New Physician* 27, no. 5 (May 1978): 17–20.

"Maggie Joins Hospice Action." *Gray Panther Network,* Summer 1978.

MANNES, MARYA. *Last Rights: A Case for the Good Death.* New York: Signet/ New American Library, 1975.

MARKEL, W. M. "The Hospice Concept." *Cancer Journal for Clinicians* 38, no. 4 (July/August 1978): 225–37.

McCARTHY, DONALD G., REV. "Ethical and Moral Aspects of Terminal Illness." Major Addresses of the Institutes on Hospices, August 1978.

———. "Should Catholic Hospitals Sponsor Hospices?" *Hospital Progress* 57, no. 12 (December 1976): 61–65.

McINTIER, SISTER TERESA MARIE. "Hillhaven Hospice: A Free-Standing, Family-Centered Program." *Hospital Progress,* March 1979, pp. 68–72.

———. "Hospices: Their Purpose and Development." Major Addresses of the Institutes on Hospices, August 1978.

McKINNEY, REPRESENTATIVE STEWARD B. "Hospice." *Congressional Record,* May 12, 1978, E2550–51.

McNAMARA, EVELYN M. "Continuing Health Care: Attention Turns to Day Care and Hospice Services." *Hospitals* 52 (April 1, 1978): 79–83.

McNULTY, BARBARA. "Care of the Dying." *Nursing Times,* November 30, 1972.

———. "St. Christopher's Out-Patients." *American Journal of Nursing* 71, no. 12 (December 1971): 2328–30.

MILLER, MARVIN. "Suicide After Sixty." *Aging Magazine,* November/December 1978, p. 28.

"A More Dignified Way to Die." *Help Age International From England* 5 (September/October 1977).

MORRISON, R. S. "Dying." *Scientific American,* September 1973, pp. 54–62.

MOUNT, B. M. "The Problem of Caring for the Dying in a General Hospital: The Palliative Care Unit as a Possible Solution." *Canadian Medical Association Journal* 115, no. 2 (July 17, 1976): 119–21.

National Hospice Organization. "Evaluation and Research Committee Summary Report." October 5–6, 1978.

———. *Preliminary Directory of the NHO.* New Haven: National Hospice Organization, 1978.

National Hospice Organization Standard and Accreditation Committee. *Hospice Standards,* August 1, 1978.

"New Haven Hospice Provides Home Care for the Terminally Ill." *American Journal of Nursing* 717, no. 74 (April 1974).

PAIGE, ROBERTA LYDER and LOONEY, JANE FINKBINER. "Hospice Care for the Adult." *Death and Dying: Challenge and Change.* Reading, Mass.: Addison Wesley, 1978.

*Palliative Care Service: Pilot Project.* Montreal: Royal Victoria Hospital, McGill University, 1976.

PIERCE, HENRY W. and WALGREN, RIPS. "Health Care, Urges Hospices." *Pittsburgh Post Gazette,* August 31, 1978.

PLANT, JANET. "Finding a Home for Hospice Care in the United States." *Journal of American Hospital Association* 51 (July 1, 1977): 53–62.

POWLEDGE, T. M, "Death as an Acceptable Subject." *New York Times,* July 25, 1978, 4:8.

RANDAL, JUDITH. "The Hospice Movement is Growing." *Arizona Daily Star,* October 13, 1978.

REZENDES, DENNIS. "Hospice: A National View." Major Addresses of the Institutes on Hospices, sponsored by the Catholic Hospital Association, August 1978.

REZENDES, DENNIS and ABBOTT, JOHN. "Hospice Movement: Way Stations for the Terminally Ill." *Perspective on Aging,* January/February 1979, pp. 6–10.

ROACH, M. SIMONE. "The Experience of an Academic as Care Giver: Implications for Education." *Death Education* 2, no. 1–2 (Spring/Summer 1978): 99–111.

ROGERS, BARRY LEGROVE. "Using the Creative Process with the Terminally Ill." *Death Education* 2, no. 1–2 (Spring/Summer 1978): 123–26.

RONES, PHILIP. "Building Design for the Elderly." *Occupational Outlook Quarterly,* Spring 1978, pp. 45–78.

ROSEL, N. "Toward a Social Theory of Dying." *Omega* 9, no. 1 (1978–79): 49–51.

ROSSMAN, PARKER. *Creating New Models of Care for the Terminally Ill.* New York: Association Press, 1977.

———. "A Prophetic Ministry to the Dying: An Interview With Edward Dobihal." *The Christian Century* 93, no. 14 (April 1976): 384–87.

RYDER, CLAIRE F. "Terminal Care: Issues and Alternatives." *Public Health Reports* 92, no. 1 (January/February 1977): 20–29.

San Diego County Hospice Corporation. *Quarterly Report: August 1, 1978–October 31, 1978,* San Diego: San Diego County Hospice, 1978.

———. *Quarterly Report: November 1, 1978–January 31, 1979.* San Diego: San Diego County Hospice, 1979.

SATCHELL, MICHAEL. "How to Enjoy Life Up to the Last Moment." *Parade,* October 16, 1977.

SAUNDERS, CICELY. "Care of the Dying." *Nursing Times* 72, (1976): pp. 1089–91, 1133–35, 1172–74, 1203–5, 1247–49, 1003–5, 1049–51.

———. "Telling Patients." Reprint, *District Nursing,* September 1965.

———. "The Care of the Dying." *Gerontologia Clinica* 9, no. 4–6 (1967): 385–92.

———. "The Care of the Terminal Stages of Cancer." *Annals of Royal College of Surgeons* 41 (July–December 1967): 162–69.

———. "The Last Stages of Life." *American Journal of Nursing* 65, no. 3 (March 1965): 70–75.

———. "The Working of St. Christopher's." Chapter contributed to *Medical Care of the Dying Patient,* Foundation of Thanatology.

———. "Training for the Practice of Clinical Gerontology: The Role of Social Medicine." *Interdisciplinary Topics of Gerontology* 5 (1970): 72–78.

———. "Treatment of Intractable Pain in Terminal Cancer." *Proceedings of the Royal Society of Medicine,* 191, no. 3, March 1963, pp. 195–97.

———. "Watch With Me." Reprint, *Nursing Times* 61, no. 48 (November 26, 1965): 1615–17.

SHAPIRO, MARY. "Legal Rights of the Terminally Ill." *Aging Magazine,* November-December 1978, p. 22.

SHEPHARD, D. A. E. "Principles and Practice of Palliative Care." *Canadian Medical Association Journal* 116 (March 5, 1977): 522–26.

SHUSTERMAN, LISA. "Death and Dying—A Critical Review of the Literature." *Nursing Outlook* 21, no. 7 (July 1973): 465–71.

SMITH, MICHAEL. "Dying Artist Breathes Life into One More Canvas." *Arizona Daily Star,* October 26, 1978.

Southwest Arizona Health Systems Agency. "Staff Analysis of the Hillhaven Hospice Licensed Home Health Agency." Tucson, Arizona, December 1978.

SPILLANE, EDWARD J. "An Analysis of Catholic-Sponsored Hospices." *Hospital Progress,* March 1979, pp. 46–50.

———. "The Hospice Under Catholic Sponsorship." Major Addresses of the Institutes on Hospices, August 1978.

Standards and Accreditation Committee Report, submitted to the National Hospice Organization Board, September 1978.

STEINBERG, MARION. "Death With Dignity." *The Journal of Connecticut Business and Industry Association* 11, no. 54 (November 1976).

STODDARD, SANDOL. "Let's Watch Our Language." National Hospice Organization, October 5, 1978, pp. 1–11.

———. *The Hospice Movement.* Briarcliff Manor, New York: Stein and Day, 1978.

"Terminal Care: Connecticut Corporation Will Build a Hospital for the Dying." *Modern Health Care,* July 1974, p. 101f.

TOZER, ELIOT. "Hospices." *Practical Psychology for Physicians,* September 1976.

TREGDE, LORRAINE. "Hospice Experience Within a Facility." Major Addresses of the Institutes on Hospices, sponsored by Catholic Hospital Association, August 1978.

TWYCROSS, R. G. "The Terminal Care of Patients with Lung Cancer." *Postgraduate Medical Journal* 49 (October 1973): 732–37.

VACHON, M. L. S. "Motivation and Stress Experienced by Staff Working with the Terminally Ill." *Death Education* 2, no. 1–2 (Spring/Summer 1978): 113–22.

VON HOFFMAN, NICHOLAS. "The Struggle to Die in Peace." *Washington Post,* May 30, 1978, reprinted by Walgren in Congressional Record, June 1, 1978.

WALD, FLORENCE S. "For Everything There is a Season and a Time to Every Purpose." *The New Physician* 18, no. 4 (April 1969): 278–85.

WALD, HENRY J. *A Hospice for Terminally Ill Patients.* Master's thesis, Columbia University School of Architecture, 1971.

WALGREN, DOUGLAS. "A Tribute to Doctor Josephine Magno." *Congressional Record,* April 4, 1978, E1642.

———. "H. R. 12358, A Bill to Amend the Public Health Service Act." *Congressional Record,* April 25, 1978.

WALKER, CYNTHIA. "Aiding the Family Through Grief and Bereavement." Major Addresses of the Institutes on Hospices, August 1978.

WEIST, V. A. "St. Christopher's Hospice." *International Nursing Review* 14, no. 5 (September/October 1967): 38.

WENTZEL, K. "The Dying Are the Living." *American Journal of Nursing,* 76, no. 6 (June 1976): 956–57.

WESSEL, MORRIS A. "To Comfort Always." *Yale Alumni Magazine,* June 1972, pp. 17–19.

WEST, D. T. "Hospice Care for a Dying Person and His Family." Paper given at First International Conference on Patient Counseling, Amsterdam, April 1976.

WEST, THOMAS S. "Approach to Death." *Nursing Mirror* 139, no. 15 (October 10, 1974): 56–59.

———. "Drug Control of Common Symptoms in the Terminally Ill Patient." *South African Medical Journal,* March 26, 1977, pp. 415–18.

WESTBERG, GRANGER. "Aiding the Family Thru Grief and Bereavement." Major Addresses of the Institutes on Hospices, August 1978.

"What You Always Wanted to Know About Hospice Care—But Were Afraid to Ask." *Aging Services News,* March 16, 1979, pp. 1–4.

WHITMAN, HELEN H., and LUKES, S. J. "Behavior Modification for Terminally Ill Patients." *American Journal of Nursing* 75, no. 1 (January 1975): 98–101.

WILL, G. "A Good Death." *Newsweek,* January 9, 1978, p. 72.

WINNER, A. L. "Death and Dying." *Journal of the Royal College of Physicians of London* 4, no. 4 (July 1970): 351–55.

WOODSON, R. "Hospice Care in Terminal Illness." In *Psychosocial Care of the Dying Patient,* edited by Charles Garfield. New York.: McGraw Hill, 1978, pp. 365–85.

WYLIE, NORMA A. "Halifax (1976)—Victoria General Hospital: A Nursing Model." *Death Education* 2, no. 1–2 (Spring/Summer 1978): 21–39.

ZORZA, ROSEMARY. "Dying With Love and Dignity." *Washington Post,* April 23, 1978, E4.

ZORZA, ROSEMARY and ZORZA, VICTOR. "The Death of a Daughter." *The Washington Post Outlook,* January 22, 1978.

# Index